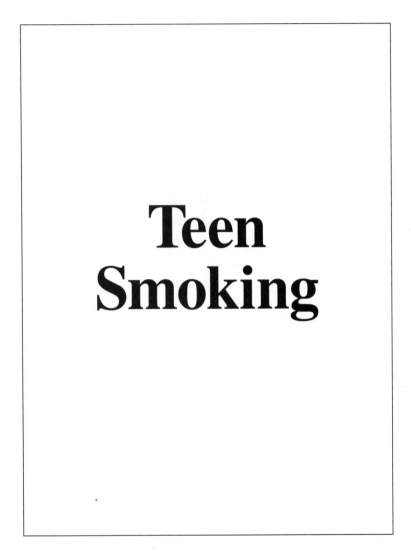

Teen Smoking

Look for these and other books in the Lucent
Teen Issues series:

Teen Alcoholism
Teen Depression
Teen Drug Abuse
Teen Pregnancy
Teen Prostitution
Teen Sexuality
Teen Smoking
Teen Suicide
Teen Violence

Teen
Smoking

by Eleanor H. Ayer

TEEN ISSUES

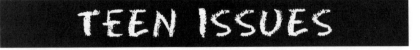

LUCENT Overview Series

Lucent Overview Series

Acknowledgments

A heartfelt thank you to Barb Wright of the Carbon Valley Library in Frederick, Colorado, for her help in tracking down many hard-to-find resources, and in leading a novice through the infinite mazes and passageways of the Internet.

Grateful acknowledgment to Sabrina Williams at the Campaign for Tobacco-Free Kids for her help in networking with several dynamic teen leaders who are active in the battle against tobacco.

Library of Congress Cataloging-in-Publication Data

Ayer, Eleanor H.
    Teen smoking / by Eleanor H. Ayer.
       p.   cm. — (Lucent overview series. Teen issues)
    Includes bibliographical references and index.
    ISBN 1-56006-442-0 (lib. bdg. : alk. paper)
    1. Teenagers—Tobacco use—United States—Juvenile literature.
2. Tobacco habit—United States—Juvenile literature.   3. Smoking—
United States—Juvenile literature.   I. Title. II. Series.
HV5745.A97   1999
362.29'6'08350973—dc21
                                                    98-25983
                                                       CIP
                                                        AC

*I would like to dedicate this book to my
friends at Alexander Dawson School
and Cornell University
in memory of my mother.*

—Madison Ayer

*The editors would like to dedicate this book to the memory of
Eleanor H. Ayer, who died shortly before its publication.*

Contents

Introduction

SEVENTEEN-YEAR-OLD Maya* doesn't smoke because she's seen firsthand what harm a lifetime of smoking can do:

> My grandma started smoking when she was 16. She's 65 now and has emphysema. Some days she can't even walk from her bedroom to the kitchen, she has such a hard time breathing. She has to use oxygen all the time, even when she sleeps. It's horrible—for her and for us. No thanks, never![1]

Those who don't use tobacco

Maya is one of the two-thirds of American teenagers who *don't* use tobacco, and she's proud of it. Indeed, for every teen who smokes, there are two who don't. The proportion is even higher among adults: Three out of four don't use tobacco products. Such figures clearly run counter to what some tobacco companies suggest in their ads: that most Americans do smoke.

Among the teens who smoke, three-quarters say they would like to quit. In a 1993 Gallup study of teenage attitudes toward tobacco, 74 percent of the twelve- to eighteen-year-old smokers said they had "seriously thought about quitting."[2] Two-thirds had tried at least once to quit, half in the previous six months. Unfortunately, only one in ten of all smokers who try to stop is successful.

Judy Swoape, who started smoking at thirteen, first tried to quit when she was eighteen. That and subsequent attempts

---

* Not her real name. This book contains quotations from teenage smokers, former smokers, smokers who hope to quit, and antismoking activists. Much of this material was recorded by the author in personal and written interviews; other quotations are excerpted from published sources. When only a first name is given, a pseudonym has been used to ensure the privacy of those who asked not to be identified.

were unsuccessful. Finally, at age thirty-nine, she was able to break her tobacco habit. "If I'd known at 13 what I know now," says Judy, "I would never have smoked that first cigarette."[3]

Tobacco use is a national, and increasingly global, health hazard, killing twelve hundred Americans daily. Yet up to 1 million U.S. teenagers begin smoking every year. In one recent four-year period, the number of teen smokers increased 7.3 percent. The Centers for Disease Control and Prevention (CDC), which has been tracking this trend, reported recently that "smoking among youth has reached its highest level in 16 years."[4]

Those who do

Just how many young people do smoke? The Campaign for Tobacco-Free Kids, the nation's largest private organization dedicated to protecting young people from tobacco use, estimates that there are more than 4.1 million smokers in this country between the ages of twelve and seventeen.

Up to 1 million teenagers begin smoking every year. Health agencies worry that the trend in teen smoking is increasing.

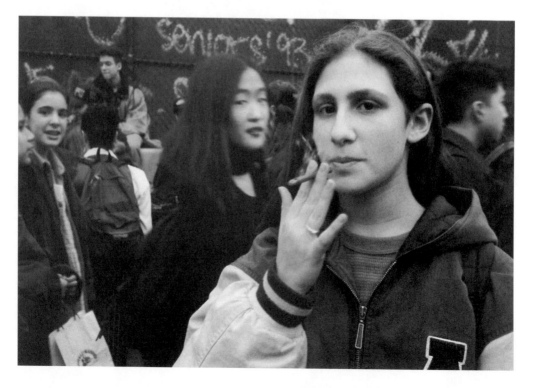

According to results of research published in *Scientific American*, "six million American teenagers and 100,000 children under age 13 smoke."[5]

David Kessler, a physician and former head of the U.S. Food and Drug Administration (FDA), has called smoking "a pediatric disease." Dr. Kessler reasons that, since nicotine addiction begins when most tobacco users are teenagers, "a person who hasn't started smoking by age 19 is unlikely to ever become a smoker."[6] The average smoker picks up the habit at age 14.5. By the time America's youth are seniors in high school, says the Campaign for Tobacco-Free Kids, 36.9 percent of them are smoking.

It's not just cigarettes they're smoking. The CDC reports that more than one in four U.S. teens aged fourteen to nineteen smoked at least one cigar in the last year. Nearly 3 percent smoked fifty cigars during that period, says an article in the *Washington Post*. At the moment, cigars are faddish among teens. But in the long run, they can be just as deadly

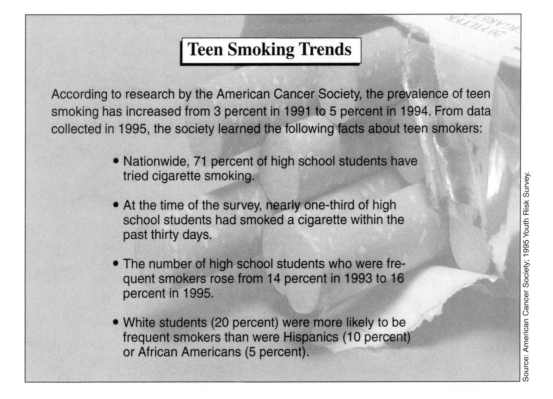

Teen Smoking Trends

According to research by the American Cancer Society, the prevalence of teen smoking has increased from 3 percent in 1991 to 5 percent in 1994. From data collected in 1995, the society learned the following facts about teen smokers:

- Nationwide, 71 percent of high school students have tried cigarette smoking.

- At the time of the survey, nearly one-third of high school students had smoked a cigarette within the past thirty days.

- The number of high school students who were frequent smokers rose from 14 percent in 1993 to 16 percent in 1995.

- White students (20 percent) were more likely to be frequent smokers than were Hispanics (10 percent) or African Americans (5 percent).

Source: American Cancer Society; 1995 Youth Risk Survey.

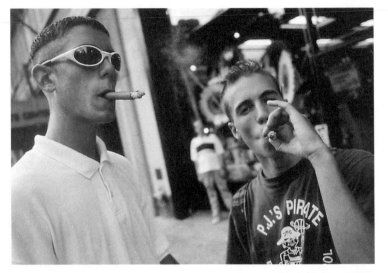

Cigar smoking is be-coming more popular among teens despite the risk of contracting cancers that are linked to this habit.

as cigarettes. Published reports have linked cigar smoking with cancers of the throat, mouth, and lungs, to the extent that cigar smokers are four times more likely to die from these diseases than are nonsmokers.

Nor is smoking the only problem. There are serious, potentially fatal, health risks from using smokeless tobacco. R. J. Reynolds, founder of the tobacco company that bears his name, chewed tobacco, and his death from pancreatic cancer has been attributed to this habit. In the nineteenth and early twentieth centuries, chewing was far more popular than smoking. Until recently, it was the domain of older men, but lately chewing has become popular among younger users. In the last decade, the major smokeless tobacco market has changed from older men to teenage boys. Today 20 percent of all high school boys (grades nine to twelve) are smokeless tobacco users; in certain western states the rate is 40 percent. Nearly three-fourths of them say they began chewing in the ninth grade or earlier.

Smokeless products come in many forms. There is the familiar pouch-type loose-leaf chewing tobacco, preferred by older men, and a softer, block form called plug. Nasal snuff, used extensively in the nineteenth century, is rarely seen now. The most popular smokeless products among teens are "chew" or "moist snuff" with brand names like

Skoal and Copenhagen, which are used orally between the cheek and the gum. One company, U.S. Tobacco, controls more than 80 percent of the market for moist snuff. The firm advertises heavily through rodeo events. Said the general manager of the National College Rodeo Finals, "U.S. Tobacco is the oldest and best friend college rodeo ever had."[7]

The dangers of smokeless tobacco are not as great to the lungs as those from cigarette smoking, but the mouth and digestive system are much more vulnerable. The surgeon general's office has stated that "the use of oral snuff can lead to oral cancer, gum disease, and nicotine addiction, and increases the risk of cardiovascular disease, including heart attack."[8] Other studies show that repeated use of oral tobacco increases the risk of cancers of the esophagus, pharynx, larynx, stomach, and pancreas. Citing reports from the CDC and the surgeon general's offices, the Campaign for Tobacco-Free Kids estimates that users of smokeless tobacco are fifty times more likely to develop cancer than nonusers.

Personality profiles of tobacco users

In Montana, where chewing is popular among rodeo cowboys, teenagers emulate their heroes by chewing snuff. By using tobacco, these kids hope to build the same image for themselves. They believe that chewing snuff will help them become more interesting and respected. Likewise, many young teenage boys smoke Marlboros to be macho and masculine like the Marlboro Man.

Low self-esteem is a common trait among teen tobacco users. Young smokers typically have little self-confidence. They take up tobacco hoping it will make them appear more mature and self-assured. Because they are uncertain of themselves, they are more susceptible to peer pressure and can more easily be "talked into" smoking. Often such feelings of low self-esteem have their source in the young smokers' living circumstances; many in fact come from dysfunctional homes in lower economic neighborhoods. They typically have few or no long-term goals and little pleasure or success in their lives. Generally, smokers are among the poorer students: 70 percent of all high school dropouts smoke.

Teen smokers often appear slightly nervous, anxious, or hyperactive—constantly in motion but without purpose. Teen smokers tend to be insecure and somewhat antisocial. Gabe, a fifteen-year-old from Indiana, fits this profile. By his own admission, he was unpopular in middle school and wanted "to do something to shut people up." That something was smoking, which he now regrets. It was a player on the volleyball team who offered him his first cigarette. "In fact," says Gabe, "that guy has become a really good friend of mine, and sometimes I tell him I have every reason to hate him because he started me smoking."[9]

In addition to being loners, teen tobacco users get in trouble more often than nonusers. Says Dr. Joycelyn Elders, a former surgeon general:

> What is notable about tobacco use is that it consistently occurs early in the sequence of problem behaviors. When a young person starts to smoke or use tobacco, it is a signal, an alarm that he or she may get involved in other risky behaviors. . . .

Smoking may be a warning sign of social problems or that a teen is engaging in other risky behaviors such as alcohol consumption or drug use.

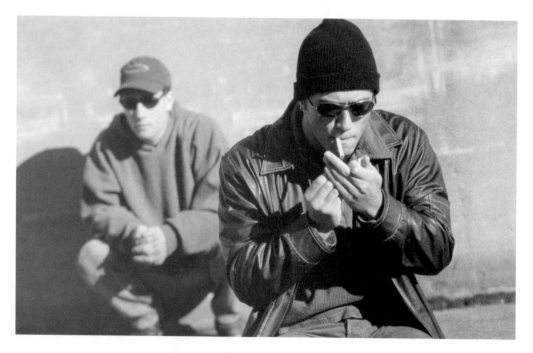

> If we can prevent tobacco use in the first place, we might have a big impact on preventing or delaying a host of other destructive behaviors among our young people.[10]

The antitobacco group Stop Teenage Addiction to Tobacco (STAT) directly relates tobacco use to other drug use. Quoting a study done at the University of Michigan, STAT says, "Illegal drug use is rare among those who have never smoked, and cigarette smoking is likely to precede the use of alcohol or illicit drugs."[11] A similar study by the National Institute on Drug Abuse reports:

> Youth between the ages of 12 and 17 years old who had smoked in the past 30 days were 3 times more likely to have consumed alcohol, 8 times more likely to have smoked marijuana and 22 times more likely to have used cocaine than those who had not smoked cigarettes.[12]

The institute further claims that binge drinking (having five or more alcoholic drinks in a row) is much higher among teen smokers than nonsmokers. In the study just cited, nearly 40 percent of smokers said they had binged in the past month, compared with only 3 percent of nonsmokers.

The Campaign for Tobacco-Free Kids, drawing on a 1994 study of cigarettes, alcohol, and marijuana done at Columbia University, calls tobacco an "early gateway drug." "The younger an individual uses tobacco, the more likely that individual is to experiment with cocaine, heroin or other illicit drugs."[13]

People who started using tobacco in their teenage years are four times more likely to use illegal drugs in their lifetime than those who did not smoke when they were young. The evidence is clear: The danger to teen tobacco users comes in many forms other than cigarettes.

1

To Smoke or Not to Smoke

IN AN AGE when most teenagers are very aware of the health hazards of tobacco, why do many still choose to use it? One young smoker from Baltimore answered that question very bluntly: "A lot of people smoke to give the finger to the world." [14]

Smoking: an act of rebellion

That frank statement reflects one of the more common reasons kids start smoking: defiance of authority. During the teenage years, young people begin to break their ties with home and become adults. Part of this process involves resisting control by their parents and other elders. Some defy authority in small ways like staying out past their curfew, others in more serious ways by breaking the law. While the purchase of tobacco products is illegal, under federal law, for people under eighteen years of age, the law is only lightly enforced. Fines against sellers are relatively small and rarely imposed, so retailers are lax in demanding identification from buyers. Smoking is therefore seen as a "safe" way for teens to rebel. Fourteen-year-old Megan from Delaware was one such rebel. Repeatedly her mother had told her about the hazards of smoking, but Megan defied her advice. "I knew she didn't want me to do it [smoke], so I did it." [15] Defying her mother gave Megan a feeling of being in control.

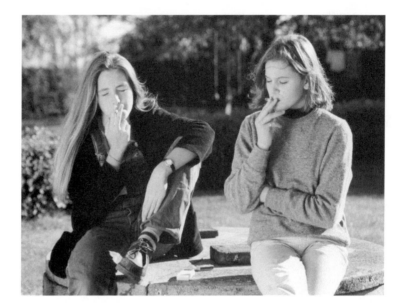

For some teens, smoking is a social activity. Most teens try their first cigarette in the company of peers.

Tobacco has an inexplicable, almost magical lure for some teenagers. Say the authors of *Teens and Tobacco: A Fatal Attraction*:

> Although smoking is fraught with hazard, cigarettes have a certain allure that no amount of reasoning seems to overcome. It's as if the more adults in positions of authority (such as parents, physicians, scientists) denounce cigarettes, the more attractive they become to certain teenagers who tend to want to mildly defy authority.[16]

Risk is part of that seductive factor. Most teens enjoy risk. The knowledge that tobacco use has harmful, potentially fatal, consequences increases its appeal. The fact that it is forbidden, by parents and the law, makes it even more alluring. To share something forbidden with friends is a step into the adult world.

Smoking: a social activity

Yet, while smoking is seen as a step toward adulthood, the 1993 Gallup study revealed that "very few teens say they smoke because it makes them feel older or because they like the way they look when they smoke."[17] They don't necessarily want to look older; more important is conveying the message, "I'm old enough to do as I please."

Nor do teens claim to smoke because of peer pressure. Contrary to tobacco companies' arguments that kids smoke because their friends push them into it, only 18 percent of surveyed teen smokers say they started using tobacco because of pressure from friends. A recent study reported in the *Journal of the National Cancer Institute* confirms this. It shows that teens are more influenced to start smoking by advertising than they are by peer pressure.

While the decision to smoke may be made independently, smoking is a social activity among teenagers. Four out of five have their first cigarette in the company of a friend. Studies show that a young person is thirteen times more apt to smoke if his or her best friend does. This relates to teenagers' need to be part of a group, to be respected by people whom they admire. For those who believe that smoking makes a person "cool," long-term health risks may seem a small price to pay.

It can't be all that bad

Many teens believe that since millions of people smoke, it can't be all that bad. Indeed, tobacco companies encourage this reasoning by running ads in which smoking is made to look natural and common. Tobacco products are available in convenience stores, supermarkets, gas stations, vending machines, and other public places. If they were really so dangerous, many teens maintain, the government would restrict or ban their sale, as it does with alcohol or marijuana. For precisely that reason, many nonsmoking advocacy groups are fighting for greater restrictions on the sale of tobacco, particularly in outlets frequented by teenagers.

Parents who smoke send the same it-can't-be-all-that-bad message. Both Reuben Salazar's mother and father smoke. "So they didn't get uptight when I started. My mom told me you can get lung cancer or heart problems, but she and my dad just kept on smoking. I figured if it was OK for them, it was OK for me."[18]

Reuben is like 65 percent of all teen smokers: He comes from a household where someone smokes. Older siblings have a particularly strong influence on younger children's

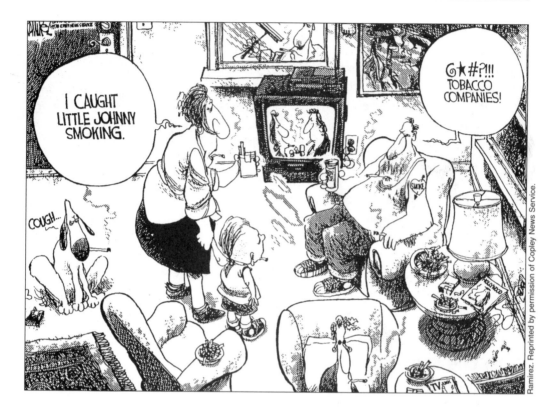

decision to smoke. When there are restrictions against smoking at home, and when community officials enforce smoking regulations, teens get a different message. They understand that smoking is harmful and illegal for people under eighteen.

Contracting the habit

Curiosity—not pressure from friends, family, or peers—is the reason 66 percent of teenagers give for trying tobacco in the first place. Most of them are lured by clever ad designers who know that teenagers are more apt to start smoking than are any other group. By age thirteen, 56 percent of all American children have tried smoking, and 9 percent are regular users. The percentages increase with each birthday. By age seventeen, 77 percent of kids have experimented with tobacco and 25 percent consider themselves frequent smokers. Of the people who will become lifelong smokers, 89 percent are addicted by age nineteen.

Ron O'Hara, who at age fifty-one was diagnosed with early emphysema, is part of that statistic. "No question, I was hooked by the end of high school. My buddies and I smoked. Yeah, we knew it was bad for us, but we didn't care. We didn't think about it. Now that it's too late, I think about it real seriously. I only wish I had back then." [19]

It doesn't take long to get "hooked." In the Gallup study of teen smokers, half had smoked their first whole cigarette by age thirteen. Within a year, they had started to inhale, and by age fifteen, half the group had purchased their first cigarettes. The average teen smoker claims to smoke eight cigarettes per day, but at least 18 percent said they smoke a full pack a day. The result: Nearly one American teen in four is a "heavy"—more than a half-pack-a-day—smoker by age seventeen.

By the time teenagers become heavy smokers, the habit has begun to control them. Four out of ten teens in the study said they smoke their first cigarette within an hour of waking up. Another quarter admitted they had trouble refraining from smoking in public areas where it was banned. Experts say that the need for a cigarette early in the day and the stress one feels when prevented from smoking are among the first signs of becoming a habitual user.

Becoming a habitual user

What leads teens from experimenting with tobacco to becoming habitual users? Partly, it's their age. The teenage years are a time when peer acceptance is very important. It's also a time of high stress, with pressure coming from all directions to be more grown up, more responsible, more mature. Some teens are pressured to do well in school or athletics. Others are caught up in romantic or sexual relationships; still others are lured by drugs or alcohol. When these pressures lead to feelings of insecurity, it is natural to look for a way to calm down, stabilize. Under such conditions, many turn to tobacco.

Simply being around friends who smoke can turn an occasional smoker into a habitual smoker. Gabe, the fifteen-year-old from Indiana who started smoking "to shut people

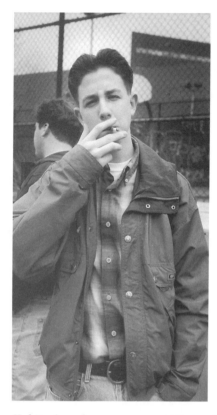

Habitual smokers usually begin smoking because of some other need: to fit in, to have something to do, or to combat stress.

up," says playing in a band and being involved with rock music contributed to his tobacco habit. Using a justification that is common among teen smokers, he says he smoked "only" to gain access to a coveted circle of friends:

> Whenever I went to concerts, there were a lot of older guys and I would have felt really out of place if I hadn't been smoking. In fact, I think the only thing I like about smoking is that it opened doors with a lot of people and gave me so many friends. I don't think I would be friends with a lot of my current friends now if it weren't for smoking 'cause it just sort of broke the ice.[20]

Many teens say they smoke because of what they call an "inner need": "It jacks me up." "It calms me down." Others like the image of a smoker—a person who, holding a cigarette, appears self-assured and in control. They want to project that image themselves. Thirteen-year-old Jimmy Igoe offers an even more vague reason for smoking:

> The main reason my friends and I smoke is it's become a habit. If I'm not doing anything, then I light up a cigarette. It gives you something to do. And if you don't have anything handy to eat or drink, it gives you a taste in your mouth.[21]

Kids who feel they have a weight problem are more specific about their reason for using tobacco. One of those is sixteen-year-old Jenny, who says:

> I've fought fat since I was in elementary school. I have this constant craving—I guess you could call it a habit—of having to put something in my mouth. For most of my life it was food or pop. Now it's a cigarette—with zero calories![22]

Jenny is part of the 40 percent of female teen tobacco users who smoke to control their weight. Among boys who smoke, one-quarter say they do it for weight reasons.

Will, an eighteen-year-old college freshman, had smoked lightly during high school, "more to be part of the crowd than anything." But he found the transition from high school to college extremely stressful.

Suddenly there was pressure from all sides. I couldn't find enough hours in the day to study, go to classes, work, eat, socialize, and sleep, so sleep was the thing I cut out. Being tired made the stress even greater. I found myself lighting up at least once an hour. I smoked to relax after classes and at night, and in the morning I smoked to get stimulated and focused before I went to class. Smoking really helps your concentration. Pretty soon—like within the first month—I had nailed down a pack-a-day habit.[23]

Most teens like Will don't intend to increase their tobacco consumption. It just happens. Six months ago they may have gone a whole day without a cigarette or chew; suddenly that's impossible. Over the weeks, as they became heavier users, they began to feel a physical need for tobacco. Before they realized it, they had become habituated. It was then that they discovered it was nearly impossible to quit.

Nearly half of female teen smokers claim to smoke in order to control their weight.

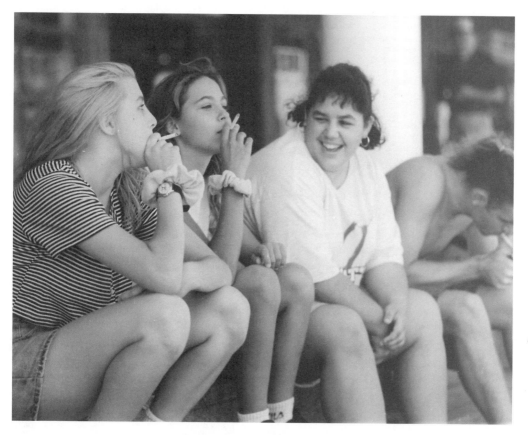

Choosing not to smoke

Fourteen-year-old Jordan, already a varsity basketball player, has many friends who smoke. He never picked up the habit himself, not only because he knows he'd be kicked off the team for smoking, but because he wants to keep his body in top condition. Jordan's concerns are not for his long-term health: "I don't think much about lung cancer or heart disease. I just want to stay in shape right now. I run five miles every day; I work out on the weights. Why would I want to mess all that up by smoking?"[24]

Some teens who cite health reasons for not smoking say they worry as much about other people's health as their own. Says Nicole:

> I hate it when you go to the mall or to a restaurant and you have to walk through a section where everyone's smoking. It just gags me. I really believe that secondhand smoke is harmful and there's no way I could do that to other people. My older sister has asthma and has a hard enough time breathing clean air. I can't imagine what it would do to her if I smoked.[25]

Overwhelmingly, teens who don't smoke say they never started because they know their parents would disapprove. "My dad would hit the ceiling," says thirteen-year-old Roscoe. And his friend Tyler adds, "My dad would hit *me!*"[26]

Teens take note

Tobacco is more harmful to teens than to any other age group. This is partly because their bodies are still growing, and developing tissue is more easily damaged than mature tissue in adult bodies. Thus teen smokers are more susceptible to developing cancer than are adult smokers or nonsmoking teens.

The lungs are particularly vulnerable. Smokers who start in their early teens may find that their lungs never develop properly and that they are haunted by respiratory problems all their lives. Teen smokers are at a disadvantage from a vanity standpoint as well, for smoking damages skin tissue and makes smokers four times as likely to develop facial wrinkles as nonsmokers.

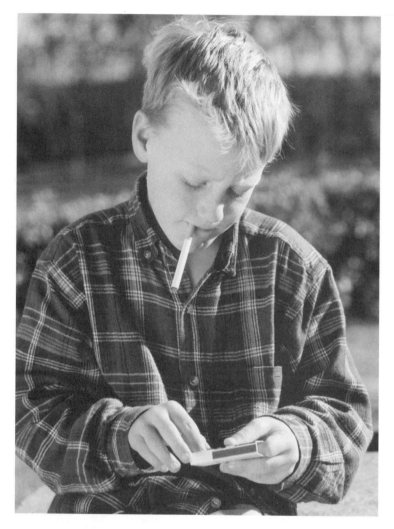

The younger a person begins smoking, the more likely he or she will smoke heavily in later years and the harder it will be to quit.

Studies have shown that the earlier a person starts smoking, the more likely he or she is to smoke heavily. Because they will ingest more of tobacco's harmful substances, habitual smokers are more apt to suffer severe health problems than are light or occasional smokers. Likewise, heavy smokers have a more difficult time quitting. It has also been found that the younger a person begins to smoke, the harder it will be for him or her to quit.

Young people should also consider their child-bearing years when weighing the risks of smoking. The publication "Tobacco Facts" notes that cigarette smoking is the single most powerful determinant of poor fetal growth in the developed world. Women who smoke have significantly more stillbirths and babies that die during the first month of infancy. Smokers' babies average 1.8 lbs. less in birth weight than nonsmokers'. [27]

Parenting problems begin for smokers even before a child is conceived. Women who smoke are three times more likely to have conception problems than women who don't. Male smokers likewise suffer fertility problems. Studies have shown that smoking reduces the speed and number of sperm cells released. The chances of those cells being abnormal is also greater among smokers than nonsmokers. Action on Smoking and Health (ASH) estimates that smoking boosts impotence by at least 50 percent.

Tanya is a rare teenager who started smoking at age thirteen, became a regular smoker within a few months, but was able to quit before she turned fifteen. "It seemed like the bad news was just coming at me from all sides," Tanya explained.

> Smokers die younger. They die horrible deaths from emphysema or lung cancer or heart disease. Even if you don't worry about the future, you can't deny that smoking leaves you physically unfit—I felt that myself after just a few weeks. Then you think you may be affecting your ability to have children in a few years, and you ask yourself, "Is it really worth it to ruin my health and the health of those around me just to keep on with this stupid habit?" I decided it wasn't. Quitting was a tough fight, but I've never regretted it. [28]

2

The Frightening Truth About Tobacco Addiction

GEORGINA DIDN'T CONSIDER herself an addict. Addicts were people who were physically dependent upon a drug. Two kids at school were crack addicts, and everybody considered them lowlifes. Some people called Georgina's cousin, Francine, a food addict. She was at least fifty pounds overweight and obsessive about eating.

So when Georgina's boyfriend accused her of being addicted to tobacco, she called him absurd. They had a big argument and didn't speak for two days. During that time, Georgina thought about addiction and about her smoking habit. It was true that she felt a craving for a cigarette after an hour or more. It was true that when she went without smoking for much of the day, she was in a bad mood. But did that mean she was addicted?

Not according to high-ranking tobacco company executives. In hearings before the U.S. Senate in 1998, most tobacco execs wavered on the question of addiction. Said Nick Brookes, chief executive officer (CEO) of Brown and Williamson Tobacco Corporation, "I wouldn't personally, in a serious debate about smoking, label tobacco as addictive. . . . What addiction, in my use of that word, means, is that people can't quit." Vincent Gierer Jr. of U.S. Tobacco added, "I would consider it more of a habit than I would an addiction." However, Steven Goldstone, CEO at

R. J. Reynolds (RJR), edged somewhat closer to acknowledging the addictive properties of his company's products: "I've always thought, and I was a smoker, that cigarette smoking is habit-forming, and I think that most Americans believe that kind of activity is addictive."[29] Senators at the hearing said these vague statements cast doubt on the executives' sincerity. The CEOs had agreed to cooperate, but were they willing to share their research about addiction in the ranks of their customers?

The truth is that tobacco company officials have known for years that tobacco is addictive. Ross Johnson, former CEO at R. J. Reynolds, was quick to acknowledge the habit-forming properties of tobacco after leaving his position at RJR. When asked whether nicotine was addictive, he answered quickly, "Of course it's addictive. That's why you smoke the stuff."[30]

What does it mean to be addicted?

The word *addiction* doesn't apply simply to illegal drugs like heroin and crack. It applies to any substance, legal or illegal, on which the user becomes physically dependent. An obsession or constant craving for a substance is an indication of addiction. The compulsive use of tobacco on a regular basis and a persistent craving after being without it for some time are definite signs of addiction. People who try hard to quit smoking but can't have become addicted.

After Georgina and her boyfriend had the argument, she decided to quit smoking for a while, just to prove to him that she wasn't addicted.

> It was terrible. On my first day without a cigarette, I was in a bad mood, which got much worse as the week went on. By the third day I was having constant headaches that sometimes took my breath away. I was popping Advil like they were M&M's, but it didn't help much. After four days, I couldn't take it any more. I smoked a cigarette, and from the first drag, the change was incredible. This wave of calm washed over me, my mood began to improve, and in a few minutes my headache started to dull. After a while I got the jitters, so I promised myself just one more cigarette—to get back in balance. Well guess what? That was the end of my quit-smoking plan.[31]

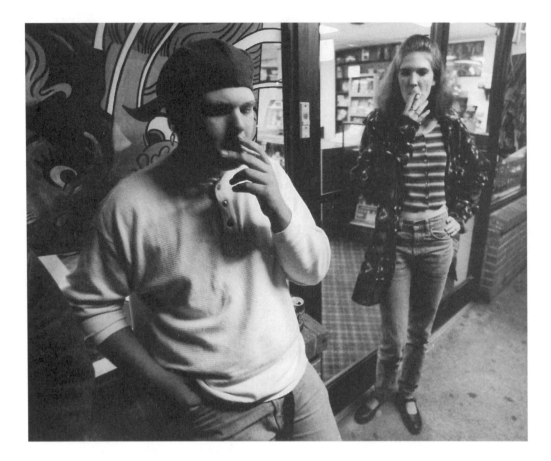

The headaches and irritability Georgina felt are called withdrawal. In the process of addiction, the body becomes dependent on a substance; if that substance is suddenly taken away, the addict suffers the mental and physical imbalance and pain of withdrawal. Georgina had become addicted to tobacco.

Regular or compulsive use of tobacco is a sign of nicotine addiction. The body's craving for more nicotine makes quitting difficult for many smokers.

Nicotine: the addictive property of tobacco

"I'm having a nicotine fit; gotta have a chew."

"I really enjoy the taste."

"It helps me concentrate."

"That first cigarette is what wakes me up in the morning."

Each of these statements is typical of a teenager who has become addicted to tobacco. Very often, addicts know the harmful effects of the substance they are using, but this awareness does not deter them from maintaining the habit. Former RJR executive Claude Teague once called the tobacco business a specialized segment of the pharmaceutical industry.

> Tobacco products . . . contain and deliver nicotine, a potent drug with a variety of physiological effects. The things which keep a confirmed smoker habituated and "satisfied," i.e. nicotine and [others], are unknown and/or largely unexplained to the non-smoker.[32]

Like Georgina's boyfriend, however, many nonsmokers don't understand the mental and physical hold tobacco has on habitual users. They don't know what it feels like to suffer withdrawal. Even many smokers don't realize what a grip tobacco has on them until it's too late. Cathy, who started smoking at fourteen, considered herself simply a social smoker. Three years later she decided to quit, but couldn't. "It was then," said Cathy, "that I realized I was addicted to nicotine and I didn't want to be. I hated myself for what I had done."[33]

Nicotine, the culprit that causes tobacco addiction, is a natural substance found in the leaves of tobacco plants. It is colorless, odorless, and oily to the touch. Nicotine is also

Nicotine is found in the leaves of tobacco plants. When nicotine enters the body it courses through the bloodstream, raising blood pressure and heart rate.

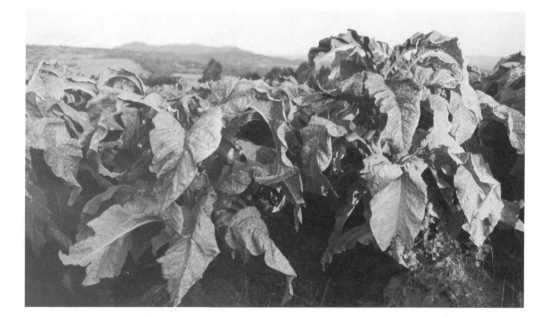

an insecticide and has even been used by veterinarians to expel worms from the intestines of large animals. Many people are surprised to learn that nicotine is a narcotic, "an addictive substance that blunts the senses and can cause confusion, stupor, coma, and death." [34]

When cigarette smoke is inhaled, or tobacco chewed, tiny bits of nicotine pass into the bloodstream. Within seconds, nicotine is racing to all areas of the body, increasing the heart rate and raising the person's blood pressure. This sudden surge in circulation and blood flow to the brain results in greater alertness and ability to focus. But nicotine also has a calming effect, for it triggers nerves along the spinal column to tell the body's muscles to relax. These physical and psychological effects last about thirty minutes to an hour, and then it's time to light up or chew again. When tobacco users are under stress, they commonly increase their nicotine intake by chewing more often or by dragging more heavily on a cigarette.

The addictive nature of nicotine is spelled out very clearly in a report titled *Motives and Incentives in Cigarette Smoking*, written by Dr. William Dunn Jr. of the Philip Morris tobacco company. "No one has ever become a cigarette smoker by smoking cigarettes without nicotine," says Dr. Dunn. And he adds, "Most of the psychological responses to inhaled smoke have been shown to be nicotine-related." [35] The tobacco industry's own actions prove this. Ninety-four percent of the cigarettes sold in the United States contain between one and two milligrams of nicotine. That means only 6 percent of the market is buying the newer brands that claim to be lower in tar and nicotine. If nicotine were not addictive, smokers would not need cigarettes with higher concentrations.

How does one become addicted to tobacco?

Nicotine addiction doesn't happen immediately. It takes from one to three years to build up a chemical dependency, which is one reason teenagers are so vulnerable. Adults who begin smoking after age twenty-one are much less apt to become permanent smokers. They have developed a circle of friends and don't need to use tobacco to look cool or to be accepted by others. In addition, it's harder for adults, with work and family responsibilities, to commit enough time to smoking to become habitual users. The increasing number of smoke-free workplaces further narrows the options for potential adult smokers. Thus it is not surprising that more than 90 percent of those who first smoke as adults give it up within a short time. Teenagers, on the other hand, are much more likely to stick with the practice until it has become a habit.

Before the body can become addicted to nicotine, it must learn to tolerate it. The learning process can be quite unpleasant, for nicotine in large amounts is considered a poison. Too much of it in the bloodstream can cause suffocation by paralyzing the muscles around the chest cavity. Travis, a habitual smoker, recalls how repulsive he found cigarettes when he started smoking:

> The first few times I tried smoking, I hated it. It left a terrible taste in my mouth and made me sick to my stomach. I threw up once. I coughed a lot. I could tell from the start that my body didn't like what I was putting into it. But I kept going because I wanted to be like my friends. Now I can't live without at least a dozen cigarettes a day.[36]

The more nicotine a person ingests, the more the body develops a tolerance for it. With new smokers, the effects of nicotine may last several hours. Among habitual smokers, the stimulation wears off in about a half hour and the craving for more begins. The more often a person smokes, the greater tolerance for nicotine the body develops. Chain smokers, who light up one cigarette after another, require an almost constant nicotine supply to maintain the "high." During sleep, nicotine is expelled from the body, so the craving for the first cigarette of the day is especially great. That first smoke has the strongest effect, for the body has been without the stimulus of nicotine all night.

"Teens slowly move from low to moderate nicotine dependency as they grow older," say Gallup study analysts. "By age 17 the first signs of high dependency begin to appear." It's not just the frequency of tobacco use that leads

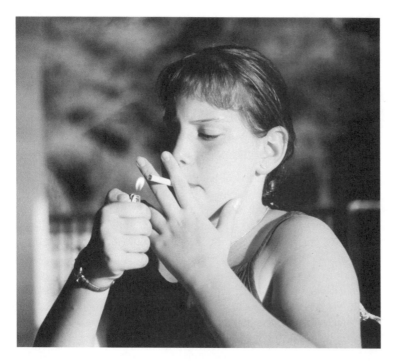

A smoker's body gradually builds up a tolerance to nicotine. The more tolerant the person is to nicotine, the more often the person will have to smoke to feel its effects.

to addiction; it's also the content of the products. Heavier smokers and chewers prefer stronger tobacco with higher levels of nicotine. "For the heavy teen smokers," say Gallup analysts, "tobacco appears to have become an integral part of their body chemistry [and] they increasingly report . . . 'I just can't help it but have to keep smoking.'"[37]

Comparing nicotine with other drugs

According to a report from the surgeon general's office, "Nicotine dependency through cigarette smoking is . . . the most common form of drug addiction."[38] This is not surprising, considering that 50 million Americans smoke cigarettes and another 6 million use smokeless tobacco products. The number of tobacco users is much greater than the number of cocaine or heroin users. In fact, an article in *Scientific American* called tobacco use a "global epidemic."[39] Nicotine, the authors noted, is at least as addictive as heroin or cocaine. Yet fewer than half the teenagers questioned by Gallup believed that tobacco products carried the same levels of danger as illegal drugs.

Nicotine is not an intoxicating drug like alcohol or marijuana. It does not noticeably alter the user's mind or behavior. But nicotine is the strongest drug in terms of dependency—difficulty in quitting—according to doctors who specialize in addiction. Most tobacco users find it extremely difficult to stop using nicotine. Repeated use leads to a chemical and mental dependency unsurpassed by any other drug. Tom Witman knows all too well about nicotine dependency:

> I was 14 when I started smoking, just for something to do. After about a year, I was having problems running track, which had always been my best sport. That was the first time I tried to quit. One day I just pitched my smokes in the trash. Didn't have a reaction, didn't feel bad when I quit. But pretty soon I was right back at it again. Second time I tried to quit was just before my 16th birthday. That time it *was* bad. I had headaches like you wouldn't believe. Started eating like a horse and put on about twenty pounds. I'd yell at people for no reason—I was bummed out all the time. That was hell, and after a month of it I started smoking again. I'll try a third time, because I really hate being hooked on tobacco. But it ain't gonna be easy, I can tell you that.[40]

The withdrawal symptoms Tom experienced the second time he tried to quit smoking are typical for a habitual smoker. Like Georgina and many other addicts, Tom had become used to a certain level of nicotine in his body, and when it was taken away, adverse reactions occurred. Nicotine is ranked third, after alcohol and heroin, for difficulties in withdrawal. The surgeon general's report puts an even blacker mark on the drug. "Nicotine dependency," it states, "causes more death and disease than all other addictions combined."[41]

Smokers' addiction affects others

An addiction to heroin is tragic for not only the addict and his or her immediate family and friends, but the rest of the community. Likewise, smokers' indulgence in their addiction adversely affects everyone around them, for they pollute the air with their habit. This pollution, described as passive smoking, comes in two forms: Sidestream smoke is produced by a cigarette left burning in an ashtray while

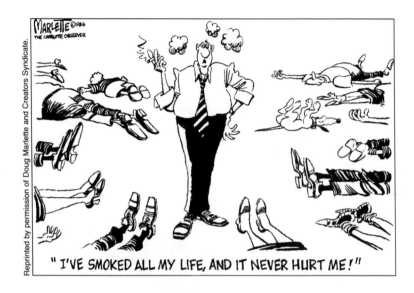

"I'VE SMOKED ALL MY LIFE, AND IT NEVER HURT ME!"

the smoker is not dragging on it; mainstream smoke is that released by the smoker upon exhaling. Because it has not been filtered through a cigarette, sidestream smoke is considered to be more harmful to bystanders.

Secondhand smoke is not just unpleasant to nonsmokers, it's significantly harmful to their health. More deaths in the United States each year are attributed to environmental tobacco smoke (ETS) than to car accidents or homicides. In fact, reports Action on Smoking and Health (ASH), "after active smoking and alcohol use, passive smoking is the third major preventable cause of death."[42] ASH estimates that passive smoking causes 47,000 deaths from heart disease every year. ETS is also blamed for an additional 150,000 nonfatal heart attacks each year. Still another 3,000 nonsmokers die each year of lung cancer that some groups attribute to ETS. And yet, heavy teen smokers say they are surprised to hear that secondary smoke can be dangerous to the health of anyone but smokers.

The effects of ETS are particularly devastating to children, who have little control over their environment. Researchers estimate that children who grow up around smokers are at twice the risk for respiratory illnesses than are those from nonsmoking homes. Like young teenage smokers, these children may also suffer from improper lung

Statistics on Secondhand Smoke

In 1993 the Environmental Protection Agency (EPA) declared secondhand smoke a human carcinogen, or cause of cancer. Approximately three thousand nonsmokers die of lung cancer each year as a result of breathing secondhand smoke. In addition, the EPA provided the following statistics:

- Secondhand smoke is responsible for the deaths of 35,000 to 45,000 nonsmokers afflicted with heart disease.

- Nonsmokers also suffer from respiratory problems caused by secondhand smoke, including coughing, phlegm, chest pain, and reduced lung function.

- Annually, secondhand smoke causes 150,000 to 300,000 lower respiratory tract infections, such as pneumonia and bronchitis, in infants and children younger than eighteen months of age.

- Secondhand smoke contains 4,000 chemical compounds, including carbon monoxide, formaldehyde, and hydrogen cyanide. Four of the chemicals found in secondhand smoke are known carcinogens, and another ten are suspected to be carcinogenic.

Source: American Cancer Society.

development and high cholesterol levels leading to heart disease. Dr. William G. Cahan, a specialist cancer surgeon, uses an alarming image to sum up the dangers of ETS: "Bringing up a child in a smoking household is tantamount to bringing him or her up in a house lined with asbestos and radon."[43]

The subject of smoking in the home raises troubling conflicts regarding personal choice and the individual liberty to use a substance that is legal but affects children's health. Any suggestions that government regulation of smoking be extended into private homes quickly encounter public opposition from many sides. Such regulation is outside the bounds of government control, but there is no doubt that the children who grow up in smoke-filled homes become the victims of addictive habits for which they are not responsible.

3

Dying a Slow Death

A CENTURY AGO, when less than 1 percent of Americans smoked, few people worried about the health hazards of tobacco. But by 1950, with half of all Americans smoking regularly, concerns began to surface. In the 1960s, when scientists showed a connection between smoking and disease, the first warning labels appeared on cigarette packages: "CIGARETTE SMOKING MAY BE HAZARDOUS TO YOUR HEALTH."

Over the years, the warning labels became more forceful: "THE SURGEON GENERAL HAS DETERMINED THAT CIGARETTE SMOKING IS HAZARDOUS TO YOUR HEALTH." Since 1984, the warnings have clearly named the principal hazards of smoking: lung cancer, heart disease, emphysema, and complications in pregnancy. Every American-produced cigarette package and advertisement carries the notice "SMOKING CAUSES . . ." followed by the name of one of the conditions. Interestingly, the 1993 Gallup study on teen smoking showed that smokers have a greater recall than nonsmokers of the messages on these labels, even though they choose not to heed them.

The facts of death for tobacco users

There is no longer any question: Tobacco is not only hazardous to one's health, it causes premature death. Some estimates indicate that half of all smokers who start as teens will die in their early sixties, fifteen years before the average nonsmoker. The Campaign for Tobacco-Free Kids, citing a report from the Centers for Disease Control and

When physicians and researchers connected smoking with certain diseases, the government required that tobacco products carry warning labels to alert users of the possible dangers.

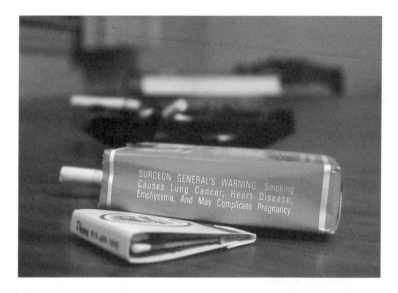

SURGEON GENERAL'S WARNING: Smoking Causes Lung Cancer, Heart Disease, Emphysema, And May Complicate Pregnancy.

Prevention (CDC), says, "More than 5 million children under age 18 alive today will die from smoking-related disease, unless current rates are reversed."[44]

Colby had heard the statistics, but he wasn't worried. At age fifteen, he had trouble relating to himself as one of the 5 million who might die early. So what if he died at sixty-two instead of seventy-seven? Old was old, and he was way too young to worry about what might, or might not, happen decades into the future. This attitude is typical of teens, who see themselves as forever young and invulnerable. Then Colby heard a statistic that made him think: Every cigarette cuts 5.5 minutes off the life of a regular smoker. Somehow that seemed more real.

> At first, five and a half minutes didn't seem like much. Then I started to think about it everytime I lit up—here goes another five minutes. When I got to the end of a pack I did the math and saw that I'd just cut two hours off my life—right then, right now. Thinking about that every time I lit a cig was what eventually got me to quit. I just hope it lasts.[45]

It was a different sort of statistic that opened Mandy's eyes. Because of dental problems, she had had many X rays by the time she was eighteen. Each time, the dentist laid a heavy lead-lined vest across her chest to protect her from the harmful rays, explaining that one should always take precautions around X rays. Mandy recalled this warning when she heard on TV that smoking a pack of cigarettes each day for one year was as harmful to your body as having one hundred chest X rays.

> That seemed unbelievable. I had been a pack-a-day smoker for at least a year. My parents and everyone else gave me grief about it, but I never listened. They all seemed like health freaks to me. But when I realized that my smoking had had the same effect as 100 chest X rays, I got really scared. I quit (for a week) and now I'm trying to quit again. I don't think kids realize how harmful cigarettes are. You see them for sale all over the place, you watch your parents and other adults smoking, you figure, "no big deal." But it *is* a big deal.[46]

Use as directed?

Most food and health products sold in the United States are subject to strict regulations by the FDA. Yet, observes the Campaign for Tobacco-Free Kids, "Tobacco poses a unique health hazard because it is the only product which kills when used exactly as the manufacturer intends." It further asserts that "virtually all new users are children and virtually all of them are addicted before they are old enough to purchase the product legally."[47]

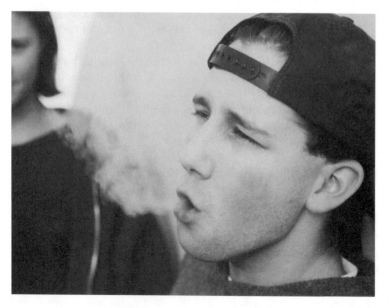

Some teens disregard the dangers of smoking because they feel the health risks posed by tobacco use will not manifest for many years.

Smoking is the number one cause of preventable deaths in America. "Cigarettes kill more Americans than AIDS, alcohol, car accidents, murders, suicides, drugs and fires combined,"[48] according to a 1994 report from the Institute of Medicine (IOM). (The IOM, which is connected with the National Academy of Sciences, studies problems in medicine and the health sciences.) Looked at another way, the IOM's data suggest that 20 to 25 percent of all deaths in the United States each year are smoking-related. Some estimates put the toll even higher. Those researchers claim that nearly 435,000 deaths a year occur from active smoking and more than 50,000 from passive smoking. Elizabeth Whelan, from the American Council on Science and Health, says smoking kills more people than "if every single day two filled-to-capacity jumbo jets crashed, killing all on board,"[49]—an occurrence that would surely bring massive changes in airline travel.

Fifteen-year-old Natasha had been smoking for a year when her grandmother, who had lung cancer, became its victim. "It was horrible to watch her die," Natasha recalls:

> In February, the doctors said she had six months to live. She only lasted four, and those months were terrible for her. She had a very hard time breathing. We kept turning up her oxygen and giving her respiration treatments to clear her airways. She had two different kinds of inhalers that she used twice a day. During the last month, she couldn't eat; she got so skinny she was just bones. The last few days she was alive, she couldn't even talk. We kept her at home till she died, but it was horrible to watch. She'd cough and cough, trying to get this junk out of her lungs, but it was so thick she couldn't. She'd just gag. I quit smoking the day my grandma died and I will never, ever touch another cigarette. I just wish I could convince my friends to do the same.[50]

Heart disease: the #1 killer

The American Lung Association (ALA) estimates that 419,000 Americans die each year from smoking-related diseases. Says the association, "Smoking is responsible for an estimated one in five U.S. deaths."[51] Researchers at the CDC blame smoking for 21 percent of the deaths from heart disease and 30 percent of the deaths from cancer.

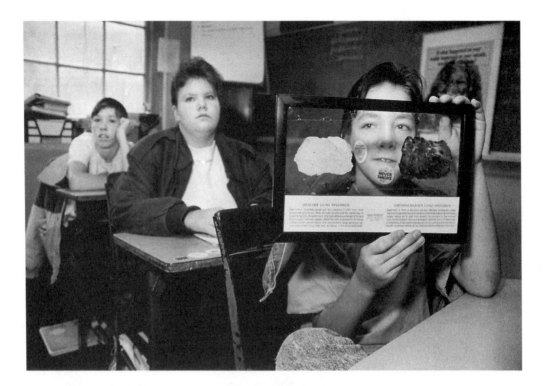

Heart disease, which is responsible for more deaths in the United States than any other illness, kills 750,000 people each year. By CDC percentages, that's more than 150,000 people a year whose lives might have been spared had they not smoked. Other experts maintain that the number of deaths is even higher. Most doctors list smoking as one of three major factors that put people at risk for heart problems. Unlike cardiac patients with a family history of heart problems or a physiological abnormality that causes high blood pressure or high cholesterol, smokers have direct control over their risk of heart disease. All they need to do to reduce that risk is quit smoking.

A student compares healthy lung tissue with lung tissue taken from a smoker. Besides breathing disorders, smoking is linked to heart disease and various forms of cancer.

Teenage smokers are in an even higher risk category. Reports from the CDC state, "The earlier the age at which one starts to smoke, the earlier the onset of coronary heart disease."[52] Since research also indicates that "the average youth smoker begins at age 13 and becomes a daily smoker by age 14½,"[53] the risk to a person who starts as a young teen is particularly high.

Why is smoking so bad for one's heart? Nicotine is again the major culprit. Nicotine increases a person's heart rate as much as ten to twenty beats per minute and raises blood pressure levels five to ten points. Such artificial stimulation puts unnatural stress on the heart. Over time, this abuse can lead to congestive heart failure, in which the heart fails to pump blood adequately.

Smoking can also cause a heart attack, where the blood vessels become blocked by clots or by a buildup of plaque, a common condition among smokers. Either situation severely inhibits the flow of blood through the body. Similar conditions can result from use of smokeless tobacco, since nicotine enters the bloodstream when tobacco is chewed.

Not only does nicotine increase the likelihood of heart disease, but it heightens the risk of other cardiovascular diseases such as strokes. A stroke is, in simplest terms, a "brain attack." Whereas in a heart attack the heart suddenly ceases to function properly, in a stroke the brain becomes unable to perform normal functions. Strokes, which are brought on by the blockage of one or more arteries that carry blood and oxygen to the brain, kill 150,000 people each year. Many others survive, but their ability to speak, walk, and breathe may be severely impaired. Tobacco use substantially increases a person's risk of stroke—doubling it according to the National Stroke Association (NSA). The good news is, says the NSA:

> If you quit smoking today, your stroke risk from this factor will decrease significantly within two years. Within five years, your stroke risk from smoking would be the same as someone who's never smoked.[54]

Cancer: the #2 killer

America's second largest killer is cancer. Like heart disease, it has been linked definitely to tobacco. Eighty-seven percent of lung cancer deaths are attributed to smoking. During the twentieth century, lung cancer became an epidemic. In 1900, when cigarette smoking was fairly uncommon, there were only a few deaths a year from lung cancer. By midcentury, when half of all Americans were smoking,

18,000 people a year died of the disease. Over the next twenty years, the figure rose to 110,000 annually, and it continues to rise.

Researchers studying this epidemic examined the lung tissue of smokers and nonsmokers. In 93 percent of the smokers' lungs, they found abnormal tissue that appeared to be precancerous. Such abnormalities occurred in only 1 percent of nonsmokers' lungs. Scientists concluded that smokers were ten to thirty times more likely to develop lung cancer than were nonsmokers.

How long and how much a person smokes have direct bearing on his or her risk for lung cancer. The outlook for

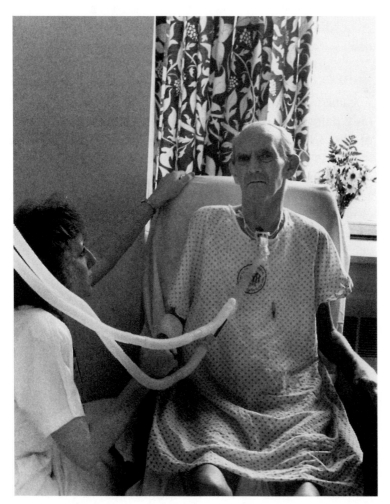

A victim of lung cancer breathes with the assistance of a machine. Smokers are ten to thirty times more likely to develop lung cancer than nonsmokers.

teen smokers is particularly grim. Says a 1994 surgeon general's report: "The risk [of dying] at age 50 for a person who began smoking regularly at age 13 is 350 percent greater than that for a 50-year-old who started smoking at age 23."[55] For women, it's even worse. Some statistics show that women who smoke the same amount as men run twice the risk of contracting lung cancer.

Lung cancer is not the only smoking-related respiratory disease. Lung damage from tobacco products causes chronic bronchitis and emphysema, as well as several other conditions collectively called "chronic obstructive pulmonary disease." Victims of these illnesses usually experience severe breathing problems and must use oxygen for years. According to the CDC, 82 percent of chronic pulmonary diseases are directly related to smoking.

Tobacco's lesser diseases

Cancer, and heart and pulmonary diseases are not the only dangers to one's health from smoking. In fact, some of the short-term diseases can be more significant to teenagers than the long-term risks. One doesn't need to become a habitual smoker to feel these effects; a cigarette every few days takes a toll on the physical fitness of an otherwise healthy person.

Smokers find that they cough and wheeze more when exercising, and that the cough raises phlegm even when they don't have colds. This is because smoking irritates the cilia, little hairs that line the bronchial tubes. When the cilia are irritated, they stop filtering foreign substances from the bronchial tubes and become covered with mucus, a thick substance that inhibits proper functioning of the lungs and normal breathing. This condition can appear within a few weeks of starting to smoke.

Even before they begin wheezing and raising phlegm, smokers may experience shortness of breath, signaling reduced lung capacity. Sixteen-year-old Jefferson noticed this only three weeks after he started to smoke:

> I started panting like a fat lady just from walking up a hill. In
> the second week of basketball season I got the flu. I've had

the flu before, but this was something else. I was out of practice for two weeks, and when I went back I was so weak I
couldn't play more than five minutes a game. It was a month
before I felt decent again.[56]

Jefferson learned the hard way that being a smoker means
colds and flus often hit harder and last longer. Whether
teens or adults, smokers are more prone to illness, particularly respiratory illness, than are nonsmokers.

Tar and carbon monoxide: the other poisons

There are many side effects of smoking that, while not
life threatening, are very irritating, especially to teenagers
concerned about their appearance. In the early weeks of
smoking, users may find themselves dizzy or nauseated.
They develop "smoker's breath," a sour smell that is repulsive to most nonsmokers. A similar smell permeates clothing and personal items. Over time, smoking stains the teeth
to an off-white or unhealthy yellow color. Food loses its
appeal, because the smoker's senses of smell and taste
have been inhibited.

The substance in cigarettes that causes these conditions
is tar, a sticky material similar to watered-down molasses.
Tar, the element that gives cigarettes their flavor, is chemically very complex. It contains three thousand different in-
gredients, some of which are poisonous. In laboratory
studies, mice that had cigarette tar painted on their backs
were more prone to develop cancerous growths than those
who did not.

Over the years, tobacco companies have marketed "low-
tar" cigarettes, but these products are far from harmless.
Many smokers believe that lower tar means lower nicotine,
but this is a dangerous fallacy. Tar and nicotine are two
separate substances. Addicted smokers tend to inhale more
deeply from low-tar cigarettes, or to smoke more often,
thus offsetting any benefit of the lower tar.

Tar and another compound, carbon monoxide, are two
of the most physically harmful substances in cigarettes.
Carbon monoxide (chemical symbol CO) is a product of

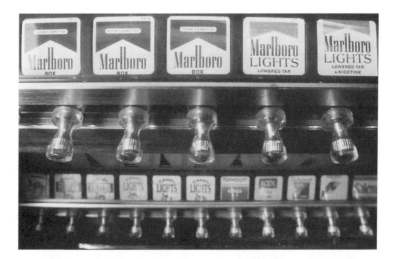

A vending machine offers varieties of regular, low-tar, and menthol cigarettes. Despite their differences, all varieties carry the same amount of nicotine, the drug that causes addiction.

incomplete combustion. As the oxygen available to a burning object is reduced, the object begins to smoke and smolder, giving off CO, a colorless, odorless gas. A cigarette, which burns slowly and with a restricted amount of oxygen, is a perfect example of a CO generator.

Carbon monoxide fumes are not specifically toxic. They do their deadly work by attaching themselves to the body's oxygen-carrying red blood cells, displacing needed oxygen molecules and thereby diminishing the oxygen supply of the person inhaling the CO. In fatal cases of CO poisoning, the victim suffers acute oxygen deprivation and essentially smothers.

The added risk of menthol

Another cigarette additive that has harmful health effects is menthol, a colorless form of alcohol extracted from peppermint oil or made synthetically. Menthol is often used in cold medications for its cooling effect on the mucous membranes. It is used for the same reason in cigarettes: to cool the harsh burning sensation experienced by beginning smokers when they inhale. Menthol itself is not harmful. But the cooling sensation it produces allows smokers to drag more deeply and hold the smoke longer; thus, they inhale more carbon monoxide, nicotine, and other harmful substances.

The 1993 Gallup study of teen smokers showed that 18 percent—a large portion of whom were black—preferred mentholated tobacco. "Among youth smokers, African Americans are dramatically more likely than Whites to smoke mentholated brands—70 percent versus 9 percent for Newport, and 12 percent versus less than 1 percent for Kool." [57]

Black smokers' preference for menthol has taken its toll in disease. The ALA reports that "African Americans smoke fewer cigarettes per day and tend to begin smoking later in life than Whites, yet their smoking-related disease mortality is higher." Figures from the American Cancer Society show that between 1957 and 1987, "the rate of lung cancer among African American men increased by 259 percent and quadrupled [400 percent] for . . . women." [58]

Sixteen-year-old Tyrone has been a menthol smoker for three years. When asked about his preference for Newports, he said:

African Americans are more likely to smoke mentholated cigarettes. The cooling sensation of mentholated cigarettes allows smokers to inhale more deeply, and black smokers have suffered higher rates of disease because of this preference.

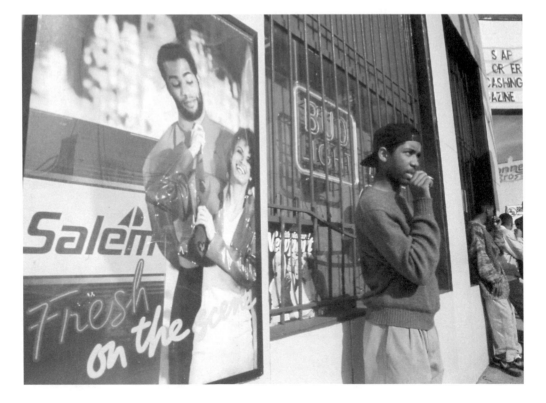

I can't exactly say why. That's the brand I started with, and that's what my friends all smoke. I've tried nonmenthols, but they're gross. They leave your mouth tasting like a cardboard box. I really like that mint taste. It's refreshing.

When asked if he was aware of the increased health hazards from menthol cigarettes, Tyrone replied, "Well, no, but I know that any kind of tobacco is bad for you. I guess it don't make much difference whether you smoke a Kool or a Marlboro. They're both likely to kill you."[59]

The Rev. Jesse Brown of the National Association of African Americans for Positive Imagery is not as casual as Tyrone in his outlook on menthol cigarettes. He feels that tobacco companies are singling out black youth with those brands. Said Brown in a speech shortly after the introduction of Camel Menthols by the R. J. Reynolds Company, "We are outraged that RJR is now targeting Black and Latino youth for death with Camel Menthols the same way the company targeted White youth for death when they introduced [Joe Camel]."[60] Quips a writer for *Tobacco-Free Youth Reporter*, a publication of Stop Teenage Addiction to Tobacco:

The tobacco industry is an equal opportunity distributor of its addictive and deadly products. . . . RJR is color and gender blind when it comes to getting their share of the market.[61]

4

Targeting Teens

EARLY IN 1998, the *Journal of the American Medical Association* published a searing attack on tobacco companies. In the editorial, editor George D. Lundberg, former surgeon general C. Everett Koop, and former FDA commissioner David Kessler declared,

> For years, the tobacco industry has marketed products that it knew caused serious disease and death. Yet, it intentionally hid this truth from the public, carried out a deceitful campaign designed to undermine the public's appreciation of these risks, and marketed its addictive products to children. . . . It claims it does not want children to smoke and then promotes advertising that appeals primarily to children. . . . By these actions, the tobacco makers have shown themselves to be a rogue industry, unwilling to abide by ordinary ethical business rules and social standards.[62]

In the same issue, the magazine ran the results of a study done at the University of California, San Diego. The subjects were teenagers who had vowed they would never smoke, not even if pressed to do so by their best friends. Three years later a follow-up study of the same teens showed that a significant number either had become smokers or were thinking seriously about starting. These teens could now name particular brands of tobacco, and some owned a promotional item from a tobacco company. The study, say its organizers, proves that tobacco ads and promotional items "entice a significant number of teen-agers to try smoking even if they were adamantly opposed to starting."[63]

In his book *Smoke Screen*, author Philip J. Hilts writes, "If it were true that the [tobacco] companies steer clear of children, as they say, the entire industry would collapse within a single generation."[64] Obviously the industry has not collapsed; indeed, it is thriving—and on revenues from people who start smoking as teenagers. Every *day*, tobacco companies spend $13 million luring the youngsters they call "replacement" smokers. This translates to $4.6 billion a year that the tobacco industry spends on advertising—an amount second only to car manufacturers.

Luring the younger market

Replacement smokers are primarily teenagers, who are known to be more apt to start smoking than any other segment of society. These kids are "replacing" smokers the industry loses each day—thirty-five hundred who quit and roughly twelve hundred who die of smoking-related causes. If the ad campaigns are successful, 2 million people will become "starters" each year. As far as the tobacco companies are concerned, the younger the better. Not only are teens more likely to become addicted than are older starters, but the younger they begin smoking, the longer they will be customers, hence the more money the industry will make on them.

Because teen smokers become such a faithful (and lucrative) market, tobacco companies have gone out of their way to appeal to them. Internal documents from R. J. Reynolds show that, as far back as 1973, assistant research director Claude Teague had teenagers in his sights:

> Realistically, if our company is to survive and prosper, over the long term, we must get our share of the youth market. In my opinion this will require new brands tailored to the youth market.

One of Teague's ideas was to develop a cigarette whose smoke was less irritating to beginners. This brand would "reduce the rate of nicotine delivery levels to accommodate the 'learning smokers.'" He proposed developing an image that would appeal to youngsters and marketing the product as an antidote to teenage "stress, . . . awkwardness, boredom,"—a means for helping shy teens achieve "membership in a group."[65] The result of the Reynolds company's image search was the phenomenally successful Joe Camel.

Other cigarette manufacturers developed their own teen brands, including U.S. Tobacco, the smokeless producer. Like Teague, it saw the value of starting kids on more pleasant-tasting brands and gradually moving them to stronger varieties. A 1985 internal memo explained, "Skoal Bandits is the introductory product, and then we look towards establishing a normal graduation process." In 1993, the company added cherry flavoring to its starter product, Skoal Long Cut. Explained one executive, "Cherry Skoal is for somebody who likes the taste of candy, if you know what I'm saying."[66] What he was saying was that Cherry Skoal was aimed at kids.

Appealing to the teenage market is nothing new among tobacco companies. As far back as 1929, Lucky Strike featured young men in its ads "breaking the chains of the

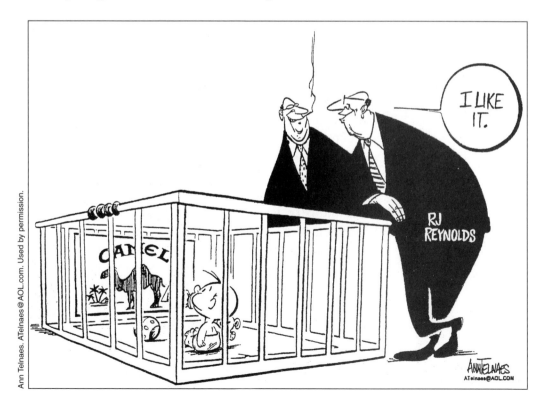

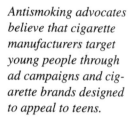

Antismoking advocates believe that cigarette manufacturers target young people through ad campaigns and cigarette brands designed to appeal to teens.

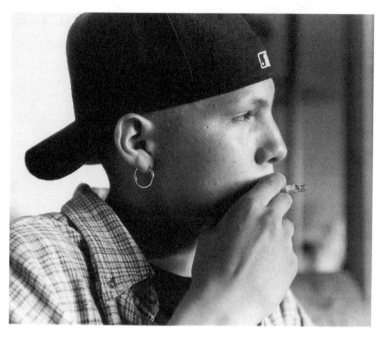

past." The ads suggested that teenage smoking was an "ancient prejudice removed,"[67] since smoking had heretofore been for men only. Throughout World War II and the 1950s, companies used cartoon characters, advertised at sporting events, produced protective covers for textbooks, and put huge amounts of money into radio advertising—a medium then highly popular among high school and college students. They even paid college students to distribute free cigarettes on campus and to help make starters feel comfortable with their new habit.

By 1964, campaigns to lure teenagers were so successful that industry leaders were pressured to address the moral implications of preying on a young market. What they did was voluntarily adopt a code that prohibited advertising specifically to people under twenty-one. Among each other, they would act as watchdogs and report violations to independent enforcement officials. The code carried a $100,000 fine for violators. But once the companies had established the code, they ignored it, and no violations were ever reported. When enforcement officials saw that they had nothing to enforce, they quit, ending the sham.

What the ads hope to convey

The point of tobacco advertising is to convince nonusers to start and lure established users to switch brands. Companies do this in a variety of ways, some subtle and some very blatant. They want to convey the message that smoking is commonplace, that many more people smoke than actually do. They want potential users to think they'll be joining a popular crowd. By showing celebrities smoking, the tobacco industry is saying subtly, "It's the cool, successful people who smoke," when actually just the opposite is true. But in the vulnerable teenage years, when one's self-image is so important, smoking helps some to build that all-important sense of self-confidence and self-assurance.

Many advertisements have definite gender association. Studies show that males, particularly teenage boys who are trying to establish independence from parents and authority figures, are lured by images of rough, rugged, sexy smokers. Teenage girls, for whom being slim, attractive, and sophisticated is important, are drawn by ads for Eve and other brands featuring women with those qualities. The ads give the impression that tobacco products help users relax in social situations. Being comfortable among one's peers is very important in the awkward teenage years.

Most cigarette ads feature young, attractive people who appear successful and popular. Critics feel that such images unfairly attract teens, who typically have low self-esteem.

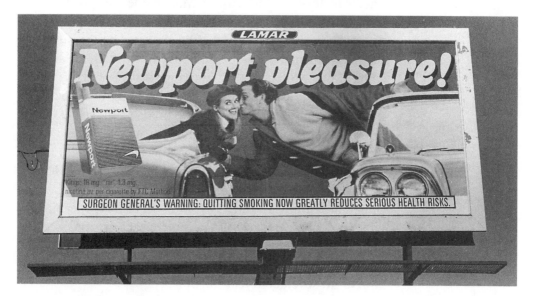

Although industry ads do not openly discuss the dangers of tobacco use—in fact, in many ads the models aren't even using the product—they aim to convince smokers that certain benefits outweigh any risks. In today's high-anxiety world, the ads say, smoking is a powerful stress reliever. At the same time, the ads often picture people in outdoor settings to imply that smoking is a healthful pastime that carries little risk. They use words like *natural* and *mild* to further enhance that image.

Tobacco's most successful ad campaigns

The tobacco companies' success at luring teen smokers is largely attributable to two enormously effective advertising programs: the Marlboro Man and Joe Camel. When 1950s research revealed that boys became smokers in attempts to demonstrate maturity and independence, the Philip Morris company developed programs to "turn rookie smokers on to Marlboro." It was trying, it explained, to create "the right image to capture the youth market's fancy . . . a perfect symbol of independence and individualistic rebellion."[68]

In the Marlboro Man, teenage boys saw the rugged, independent individual that many of them wanted to be. Likely the most successful and longest-running ad campaign in tobacco history, the Marlboro Man made his product the world's largest-selling cigarette, capturing 26.5 percent of the smoker market. Few kids who are lured by the image of the independent cowboy realize that the very first Marlboro Man, David Millar, died of smoking-related emphysema.

After nearly two decades of allowing Marlboro to dominate the youth market, R. J. Reynolds launched its own youth ad campaign, which transformed the logo of a stodgy, low-selling brand from a yellow-brown silhouette of a camel into one smooth cartoon character. Launched in February 1988, the campaign featuring Joe Camel catapulted Reynolds's Camels from 3 percent of the market share to 13 percent (overall) in a three-year period. Among teen smokers, the percentage shot to 33. Unfortunately the largest group of Camel-loving teens was the youngest, the twelve- to seventeen-year-olds.

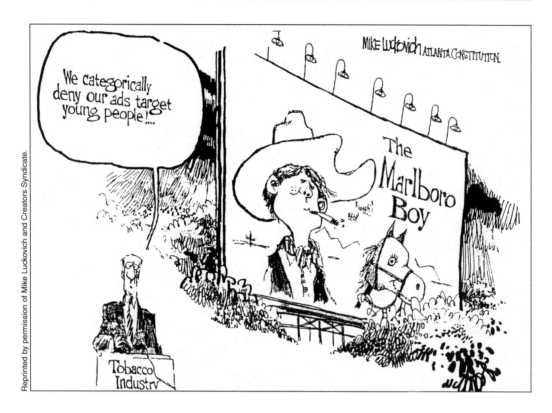

In the environment created by these ad campaigns, Marlboro came to claim 53 percent of the teen cigarette market, with Camel gaining rapidly at 16 percent. This success is tied unquestionably to the ads for these brands. "When asked about advertised brands," the Gallup study reported, "Camel and Marlboro are the ones teens most likely will name first."[69]

The enticement of advertising

The biggest enticement for teens to buy tobacco is advertising. Results of a recent study in the *Journal of the National Cancer Institute* showed that "teens are more likely to be influenced to smoke by cigarette advertising than they are by peer pressure."[70] A similar study reported by the Campaign for Tobacco-Free Kids showed that "teenagers are three times more sensitive to tobacco advertising than [are] adults."[71] The 1993 Gallup study revealed that "87 percent of the teens interviewed could recall one or more tobacco company's advertising they had seen recently" and "half could identify by sponsor at least one of four tested slogans."[72]

Oftentimes, the more subtle the message, the more effective the ad. The Joe Camel campaign didn't stress good taste or low price. It implied that people who smoked Camels would be part of a smooth, fun-loving crowd. Other brands use this strategy, as well. Says sixteen-year-old Shantel, a Newport smoker, "I liked what I saw in Newport ads. They showed the kind of people I wanted to be, doing the kinds of things I wanted to do. I felt closer to the people in the Newport ads than any of the others."[73]

Of course the ads are deceptive. Much of what they imply is false: Good friends are not determined by the brand of cigarettes they smoke; smoking will not turn an insecure, unpopular teenager into a Marlboro Man; discontented people don't begin to enjoy life simply because they take up smoking. And the ads omit the many downside factors of tobacco use: They don't reveal smokers' yellow teeth, bad breath, and hacking coughs; they don't point out the hundreds of dollars a teenager spends on cigarettes every year. Being aware of cigarette companies' deceptive advertising is one of the first steps in breaking the myth about the joys and benefits of smoking.

Premiums and promotions

Premiums such as tobacco company giveaways are another effective means of enticing kids to smoke. About half the smokers in the Gallup study said they had received promotional items like clothing, sports gear, and CD players bearing tobacco company logos. Even one out of four non-smokers had such items. Tobacco companies prefer this type of advertising because it allows them to put their logos into consumers' hands without the distraction of the surgeon general's health warnings. Young people take the products to school or to youth-oriented activities where tobacco advertising is otherwise banned.

The industry reaches its audience by mailing flyers or catalogs from which company coupons like Camel Cash can be used to purchase logo gear. Advertising departments have compiled huge lists of teenagers, both smokers and nonsmokers. "The Philip Morris mailing list," say the authors of *Teens and Tobacco* "had 26 million names in 1993, about 1.6 million of them American teens."[74]

In recent years, more than 40 percent of the industry's advertising budget has gone into so-called value-added promotions. These promotions include reduced-priced "introductory" packs, money-off coupons that can be redeemed toward future purchases, and "buy one get one free" programs. Some companies offer extra cigarettes in every package; others attach free "bonus" items to every pack. For cash-strapped teenagers, these offers are powerful enticements.

Another enticement is free samples. A quarter of the teen smokers in the Gallup study said they had been given free samples by company representatives. Each year, tobacco companies give away more than $100 million in samples, which are theoretically restricted to the adult market. Although that may seem like a lot to give away, the return in revenue from just one person who becomes a lifelong smoker can total more than $50,000.

Who gets tobacco's advertising dollars?

In years past, tobacco companies spent as much as 46 percent of their ad budgets on magazine advertising. But in recent years, due to the success of promotions and other forms of advertising in luring the teenage market, magazine advertising has dropped to less than 10 percent. The magazines that still run tobacco ads are primarily those with large teenage readership: *People*, *TV Guide*, *Sports Illustrated*, *Jet*, etc. New laws regarding advertising to the teen market are likely to change this practice, however.

Another medium affected by the new regulations will be billboard advertising, which once got up to 10 percent of the tobacco industry's ad money. On billboards, it was easy for companies to claim they were not targeting teens, particularly when the models used were plainly adults. Although warning labels were required, they were run in the

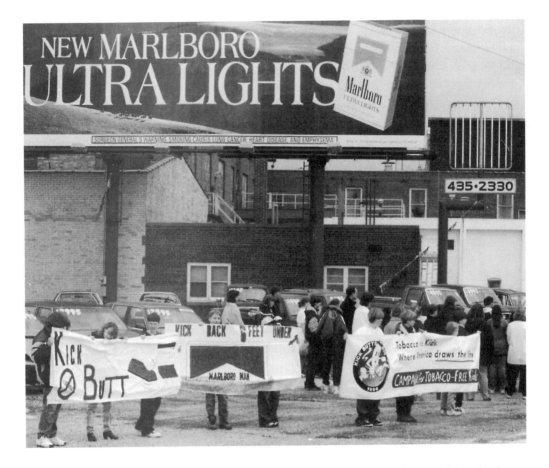

Cigarette billboards are highly visible to teens, and the required warning labels are typically small in comparison to the ads. Here, beneath such a billboard, young people protest against the smoking habit.

lower corners where they were often obscured by the huge pictures on outdoor advertising displays. Under the new regulations, billboard advertising may be banned altogether because it is impossible to control teenagers' exposure to it.

Tobacco sponsorship of sporting events may likewise die under government regulations. In this form of advertising, as with logo gear, warning labels are not required, which makes sports a friendly forum for tobacco manufacturers. One of the most insidious aspects of tobacco sponsorship is the implication that athletes support smoking and that they smoke themselves. With the teenage worship of athletes that exists in our society, there is little doubt that this type of advertising targets teens. Two of the major sports backed by tobacco money are rodeo, sponsored by the smokeless company U.S. Tobacco, and auto racing, where Winston (R. J. Reynolds) is a prominent backer.

Teenage buying practices

Even if kids aren't fans of tobacco-sponsored sporting events, don't receive direct-mail ads, and don't see magazines that carry cigarette ads, they are heavily exposed to tobacco products in gas stations and convenience stores. Usually the tobacco racks—called point-of-purchase displays—are directly beside the register, in easy view of all customers. This placement is no accident; tobacco companies pay retailers large sums—up to 7 percent of their ad budgets—for this prime space. Money for point-of-purchase space is well spent by tobacco companies. The 1993 Gallup study showed that 54 percent of teenagers buy their tobacco products at convenience stores and 29 percent at gas stations. Younger teens, who fear being asked for identification, more often buy from vending machines. Only 8 percent in the study group bought from other teens. Most agreed that they had "no problem" purchasing tobacco products, even though the legal age is eighteen. Says James, a seventeen-year-old smoker:

> Some of my friends bought fake IDs but I think that's a waste of cash. I've never been asked for ID and I've been buying for more than two years. But I don't press my luck. I never buy cartons. Buying packs is more expensive, but in eight months I'll be able to buy legally anyhow.[75]

James is one of the two-thirds of American teens who say they've never been turned away from a tobacco counter. "Nearly all teen smokers have bought a pack of cigarettes at least once," reported the Gallup study. "Four in ten have bought a carton at least once. One teen in five has bought 'loosies'—single cigarettes sold out of the pack by vendors."[76]

The tobacco companies' highly successful advertising campaigns, combined with many retailers' lax enforcement of the eighteen-year-old age requirement for purchasing tobacco, resulted in tremendous brand loyalty among teenagers. Three of the top six cigarette brands—Marlboro,

Newport, and Camel—are among the most heavily advertised. Collectively they make up a third of all cigarette sales. But in the teenage market they make up well over three-quarters of sales. Unfortunately a large part of this product loyalty is due to specific child-oriented advertising developed by tobacco companies over the last two decades. "Eighty-six percent of children who smoke, smoke the most heavily-advertised brands," reports the Campaign for Tobacco-Free Kids. "Tobacco advertising works," it concludes, "and has its greatest impact on children." [77]

5

The Big Winners

ON MAY 12, 1994, a box filled with four thousand pages of secret internal documents from the Brown and Williamson Tobacco Corporation (B&W) and its parent company, British American Tobacco, appeared on the desk of Professor Stanton Glantz in the Cardiovascular Research Institute at the University of California, San Francisco. The return address read only "Mr. Butts." These documents contained proof of what antismoking activists had long suspected: Tobacco companies were intentionally withholding information from the public and the scientific community concerning the harmful effects of tobacco. Professor Glantz and his colleagues analyzed the thousands of pages of documents and at last made public their report in a book titled *The Cigarette Papers*, which, they say, contains

> overwhelming evidence of the irresponsible and deceptive manner in which B&W has conducted its tobacco business. . . . For more than thirty years B&W has been well aware of the addictive nature of cigarettes, and in the course of those years it has also learned of numerous health dangers of smoking. Yet, throughout this period, it chose to protect its business interests instead of the public health by consistently denying any such knowledge and by hiding adverse scientific evidence from the government and the public, using a wide assortment of scientific, legal, and political techniques.

> The documents also demonstrate that B&W's conduct was representative of the tobacco industry generally. B&W acted in concert with the other domestic tobacco companies on numerous projects, the most important of which were specifically

designed to prevent, or at least delay, public knowledge of the health dangers of smoking and protect the tobacco companies from liability if that knowledge became public.[78]

The Big Six

Brown and Williamson is the nation's third largest tobacco producer, and its parent company, British American Tobacco, is the second largest in the world. B&W controls approximately 11 percent of cigarette sales in the United States, ranking behind R. J. Reynolds at 28 percent and the leader, Philip Morris, at 43 percent. These and the three smaller American tobacco companies earn approximately $45 billion per year. Out of those earnings, in a recent "bad" year, the Big Six showed a combined profit of $5.2 billion—just from U.S. sales.

Philip Morris, which began producing cigarettes in London in 1854, today manufactures the world's largest-selling cigarette: Marlboro. In some twenty-five countries, Philip Morris controls at least 15 percent of the cigarette market,

Philip Morris manufactures and sells Marlboro, the world's most popular brand of cigarette. The Marlboro Man campaign was very popular with teen smokers in the 1960s, and it continues to attract young people to the habit.

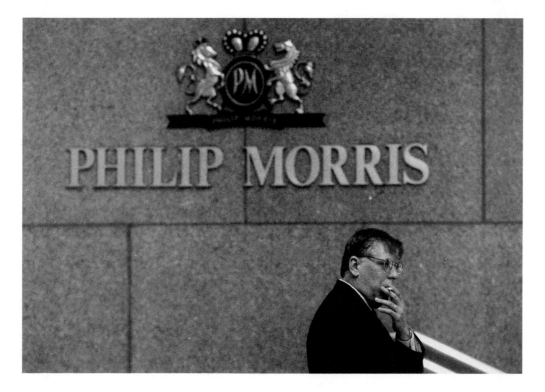

with brands such as Benson & Hedges, Merit, Virginia Slims, and Players (popular in Canada and other commonwealth countries).

Not far behind in market share is the R. J. Reynolds Tobacco Company, founded by Richard Joshua Reynolds in 1874 as a maker of chewing tobacco. By 1887, from its factory in Winston, North Carolina, Reynolds was marketing eighty-six brands of chewing tobacco, in an age when chewing was far more popular than smoking. In the early 1900s, responding to an increasing demand for cigarettes, Reynolds developed Camel, packaged with a rather unattractive picture of a circus animal. Today, Camel, a particular favorite of teen smokers, is one of the strongest selling RJR brands, along with Winston, Salem, Doral, Vantage, and others.

The British American Tobacco Company became "American" in 1927 by acquiring the small firm of Brown and Williamson and turning it into the number three player in the American tobacco game. Among B&W's biggest-selling brands are Kool, Richland, and Capri. Close behind B&W, holding 7 percent of the market each, are American Brands and Lorillard.

Unlike the giants, who have huge nontobacco holdings such as Philip Morris's breweries and R. J. Reynolds's food companies, American Brands is the only U.S. tobacco manufacturer whose sales are still primarily from tobacco products. Although American Brands does not have a cigarette on the top ten American list, it does produce such popular brands as Carlton, Tareyton, Lucky Strike, and Pall Mall. Its close competitor, Lorillard, manufactures the number five brand in the United States, Newport. Liggett and Myers, which controls 2 percent of the American cigarette market, is best known for the L&M and Eve brands.

Smoking: an American habit

Tobacco is an American product, named by the natives who met Christopher Columbus when he arrived on the continent. Using a long wooden tube called a tobacco, these people inhaled through their noses the smoke from the leaves of a species of plants called *Nicotiana*. Alternately they rolled the dried *Nicotiana* leaves in corn husks and inhaled the smoke through their mouths. Within a hundred years, the tobacco habit had spread to Europe and from there to the rest of the world. The first cigarettes were harsh-tasting, and people were deterred by the bitter jolt of nicotine they received upon inhaling. John Rolfe, the English colonist who settled in what is now Virginia and married Pocahontas, responded to the need for a more pleasant cigarette by perfecting a milder tobacco. For three hundred years, people smoked or chewed pure tobacco. But by 1950, in response to increasing health worries associated with smoking, manufacturers were soaking tobacco leaves in additives and turning out filtered cigarettes to create a "safer" product.

At the same time, their marketing departments were luring an entirely new group of smokers: teenagers. By the mid- to late 1960s, their success was apparent: The greatest increase in smokers was in the sixteen- to eighteen-year-old age group. The Marlboro Man soared in popularity among high school and college males. Lucky Strike began a teen campaign based on the slogan, "Luckies separate the men from the boys, but not from the girls."[79] For young ladies, Philip Morris introduced Virginia Slims in 1967, and within six years the number of teenage girls who smoked had doubled. Other manufacturers followed this feminist theme, and thus Eves, Silva Thins, and other "ladies'" brands were introduced.

Tobacco industry in denial

Throughout their campaign to attract teen smokers, American cigarette manufacturers made no acknowledgment of tobacco's harmful effects. Yet, since the early years of the century, when smoking first became popular, tobacco companies had suspected the dangers. In *The Gilded Leaf*, a history of the R. J. Reynolds Tobacco Company, coauthor Patrick Reynolds (R. J.'s grandson) writes:

> For many years before 1911, R. J. had believed cigarettes were harmful to health; in particular, that the paper wrapper

caused problems when it burned. Others in the company thought this was nonsense and cited the public's obvious appetite for cigarettes as reason enough to manufacture them.[80]

This practice of giving the public what it wants, regardless of the consequences to people's health, has dominated the thinking of tobacco companies through the years. In the 1940s, writes Philip J. Hilts in *Smoke Screen*, industry representatives ordered tests to determine the toxicity of tobacco smoke and the level of irritation created by the tars. One scientist's tests involved putting a single drop of the extract in rabbits' eyes. Reports Hilts:

> He had to stop the project after finding that a single drop was so toxic that it caused massive sores and the complete loss of the eye. He said it was the most toxic substance he had ever seen.[81]

Taking drastic action

The results of these tests were reported to tobacco companies, but it took another decade before signs of danger began to reach public awareness. *Reader's Digest*, which is today an openly antismoking magazine, ran its first critical article in 1952, titled "Cancer by the Carton." A year later a report in the journal *Cancer Research* telling of the tumor-producing effects of smoke condensate made its way into national newspapers. The public began to worry, and tobacco execs huddled for a crisis meeting in New York. The reports, they acknowledged, were "extremely serious" and "worthy of drastic action."[82]

Quickly the companies launched massive public relations campaigns to offset the disturbing news coming from the research labs. They formed the Tobacco Industry Research Committee (TIRC), whose major purpose was to counter claims that tobacco use was hazardous to human health. TIRC launched its own studies, but it reported none of the harmful conclusions that its scientists found. In their advertising, tobacco companies began to downplay the stress-relieving "benefits" of smoking, fearing that critics might now use such claims to support the charge that tobacco is addictive.

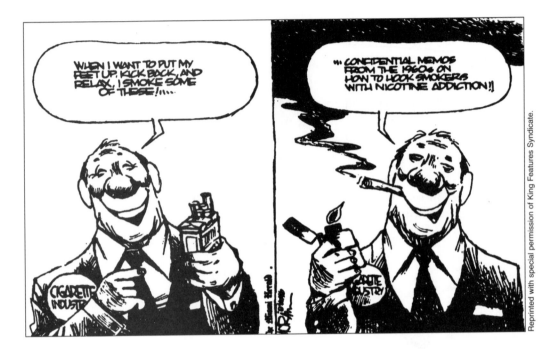

By the early 1960s, scientists had identified the most harmful properties in tobacco smoke. Their reports at last prompted the government to take a stand. In 1964, Surgeon General C. Everett Koop announced a link between smoking and lung cancer. Two years later, every package of cigarettes was required to carry a warning label, and by 1971, cigarette ads had been banned from TV and radio.

As more data were revealed, nonsmokers became vocal about the danger they perceived in secondhand smoke. Even though there was not yet proof of this danger, people started demanding smoke-free workplaces and nonsmoking sections in restaurants and other public areas. Their efforts began to pay off in 1975 with the passage in Minnesota of the first laws stipulating designated areas for smoking.

Tobacco companies exposed

The scientific revelations were accompanied by a greater public demand for the truth from tobacco companies about the nature of their products. But the companies steadfastly thwarted such requests by refusing to reveal their internal documents, their research, or other findings on which policy was based. The companies' top executives continued to claim that there was no positive proof that smoking caused cancer or heart disease. They maintained that smoking was not addictive and that people chose to smoke of their own free will. They further insisted that they were "committed to determining the scientific truth about the health effects of tobacco, both by conducting internal research and by funding external research."[83]

The insincerity of these claims was exposed in 1994, when Professor Glantz and his colleagues made public the Brown and Williamson documents that had been supplied by "Mr. Butts." The tremendous furor and upheaval that followed resulted in an investigation by the FDA, and lawsuits were filed against the major tobacco companies. The B&W reports denied that manufacturers manipulated nicotine levels to keep smokers addicted. However, they did state that "most are adding chemicals such as ammonia to increase the potency in cigarettes,"[84] ammonia being a chemical that spurs the delivery of nicotine to the body.

A flood of lawsuits

In addition to the damning evidence, a former B&W executive accused his boss of lying to Congress by claiming he did not believe nicotine was addictive. Furthermore, said the former exec, "company lawyers hid potentially damaging scientific research and . . . the company continued to add chemicals to cigarette mixtures, even after being informed that the chemicals were unsafe."[85]

These disclosures brought another flood of lawsuits by individuals, or their families, whose health had been damaged by smoking. Fearing that agreeing to out-of-court settlements would imply guilt, the companies steadfastly refused to settle, spending whatever it took to win their cases. And since most individuals were financially unprepared to battle the mighty corporations, the tobacco companies prevailed.

Following the initial lawsuits, a new round of litigation began: class action suits, where hundreds of smokers, former smokers, and family members united to fight the tobacco companies. Showing a confidence based on past successes, Philip Morris executive Geoffrey Bible announced, "We expect to prevail in all the class-action suits and underlying claims." He added with typical self-assurance, "You must remember, we have never lost a case." [86]

The FDA rule

The class action suits, the increasing public outcry, and the ongoing health revelations of the 1990s at last prompted action by the FDA and the federal government. Thus far, tobacco had been exempt from FDA regulations, for it was considered neither a food nor a drug. Additionally, it had been on the market so long that it had "grandfather" status, which protected it from regulation. Noted the *Wall Street Journal*, "a product believed to be responsible for 425,000 deaths each year got less government oversight of its contents and marketing than [did] ice cream." [87] FDA commissioner David Kessler was particularly outraged by tobacco's impact on young people.

> This epidemic of youth addiction has enormous public consequences. A casual decision at a young age to use tobacco products leads all too often to addiction, serious disease, and premature death as an adult. [88]

The FDA responded by drawing up rules to govern the manufacture and sale of tobacco products, particularly as they affected young people. Among the proposed provisions were bans on cigarette sales through vending machines, self-service displays, and the distribution of free samples. The FDA wanted to end sponsorship of sporting events by tobacco companies and the printing of tobacco brand names on clothing or other products attractive to teenagers. No tobacco ads were to appear within one thousand feet of schools. All outdoor ads and those in teen publications must be text only and run in black-and-white. The FDA proposed that retailers be required to verify the ages of any tobacco purchasers who appeared to be under twenty-seven.

The FDA rule was approved by President Bill Clinton on August 23, 1996. Said former surgeon general C.

Everett Koop shortly before its approval, "The tobacco companies are clearly adversaries not only of the public health community, but also of the very health and life of the American people, and we need to make that even clearer." [89]

The goal of the FDA rule, said Clinton, was to reduce youth tobacco consumption by 50 percent over a seven-year period. The Campaign for Tobacco-Free Kids called it "the first meaningful national policy in history to limit kids' access to tobacco and prevent the tobacco industry from marketing its deadly products to our children." [90]

Not surprisingly, the proposed FDA rule was immediately challenged by the tobacco companies. Battles raged well beyond the 1997 date when the regulations were to have taken effect. In an effort to sway politicians, "tobacco interests pumped $4.5 million into the coffers of

A flight attendant discusses her class action lawsuit against the tobacco industry during a press conference. Her suit maintains that flight attendants suffered illnesses caused by secondhand smoke.

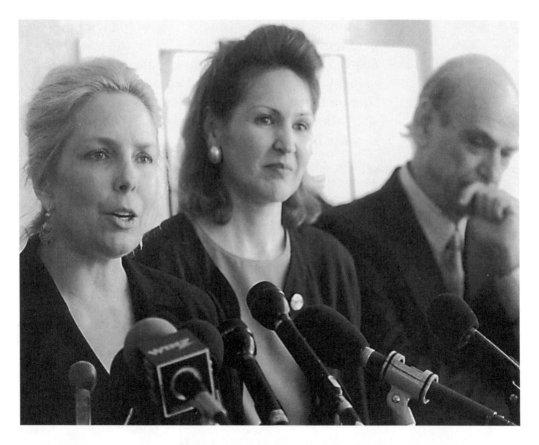

federal candidates and national political parties in 1997," reported the *New York Times*, "an industry record for a non-election year." But this time, money failed to talk as it had in the past. "In a twist," added the *Times*, "as the industry gives additional money to federal candidates and to the national parties, it finds itself with fewer and fewer friends."[91]

The controversy continues

Although the tobacco legislation remains unsettled, the industry has finally been forced to admit that smoking is harmful. In the future, the exposure of children and young adults to tobacco advertising is almost certain to be severely restricted: no more sponsorship of sporting events or use of cartoon characters such as Joe Camel, which appeal to children. Nicotine will likely be regulated by the FDA, but the agency's powers will be monitored and subject to various external controls. These complications raise questions as to whether nicotine levels will actually be reduced. One particularly controversial point is the tobacco industry's insistence that any settlement include a provision protecting the companies from further class action suits. An editorial in the *Journal of the American Medical Association* addresses this point:

> The tobacco industry has intentionally designed and marketed addictive, lethal products and deliberately hidden their well-known risks. These actions are morally reprehensible. Yet, the tobacco makers have the shamelessness to ask to be excused from liability for their informed and deliberate actions. How would we respond if the makers of cars knew their gas tanks would explode and their brakes were defective, had hidden these flaws, marketed these vehicles, lied when caught, and then made a similar request? To allow any industry to continue such acts without restriction . . . would be irresponsible in the extreme.[92]

Congress and the tobacco industry lawyers are far from reaching a settlement. "What is left of the [FDA] agreement once it has been through the Washington wringer," noted one observer, "has yet to be determined."[93]

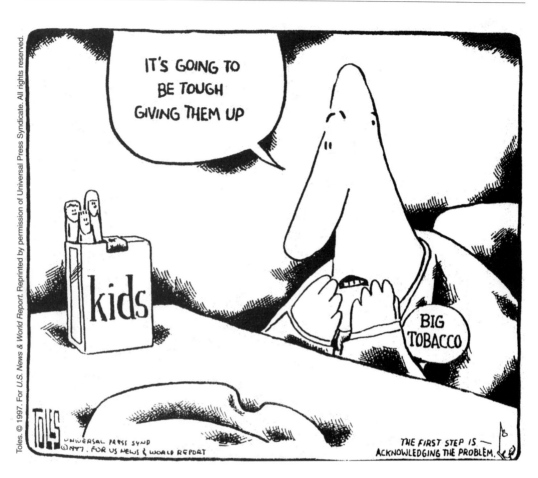

As the controversy rages, teens across America are taking a stand against the tobacco giants. Fifteen-year-old Nicole Gallegos from Denver traveled to Washington, D.C., during the tobacco settlement debate to offer testimony to members of the House of Representatives. Said Gallegos:

> We [students] believe that tobacco companies are nothing less than drug dealers in our neighborhoods, killing the American people to make a profit without any remorse. . . . We are making a stand today. We invite Congress to join us to stop the addiction.[94]

6

When It's OK to Be a Quitter

"THE MAJORITY OF teen-age smokers already have found it desirable but difficult to quit," reported the 1993 Gallup study on teen attitudes toward smoking. "Eight in 10 believe they could quit smoking if they made the decision to do so, but other findings suggest this assumption may often be illusory." [95]

The easier-said-than-done truth about quitting smoking was quickly confirmed by other teens in the Gallup study. Fully half the smokers interviewed admitted that they had made "a serious attempt to stop," but had failed. Two-thirds said they would like to quit, but had not. "Smoking becomes not a choice, like working out, or a benign habit, like eating chocolate, but an addiction," say the authors of *Teens and Tobacco*. "Only one in ten [teens] who try kicking the addiction later on [in their lives] ever succeed." [96]

Government efforts to help kids quit

Perhaps the greatest tragedy of tobacco addiction is that most teen smokers reach a day when they deeply regret their choice. Seven out of ten in the Gallup study said they would not start again if they had it to do over. A quarter of teen smokers admitted, "I just have to keep smoking." [97]

Helping kids to keep from making a decision they may later regret was one of the reasons the government cited for becoming involved in the tobacco battle. Citing studies that showed teen smoking drops about 7 percent for every

10-cent increase in the price of a pack of cigarettes, Vice President Al Gore favored raising cigarette prices by $1.10 per pack over a five-year period. The Gallup study supported Gore's proposal, for three-fourths of the smokers questioned said that an increase of $1 to $2 per pack would make them "consider some form of smoking cessation activity."[98] Occasional smokers said they would quit at once.

For decades prior to its stand in the mid-1990s, the government did little to make or enforce strict tobacco regulations. Kids acknowledge that they don't take tobacco warnings seriously. One reason, they say, is the fact that tobacco products are still legal. If they were that harmful, they reason, the government would have outlawed them as it has cocaine or heroin. Another reason is the government's weakness in enforcing its ban on sales to minors. As a result of the recent congressional action, that laxity should change. In an increasing number of states, a photo

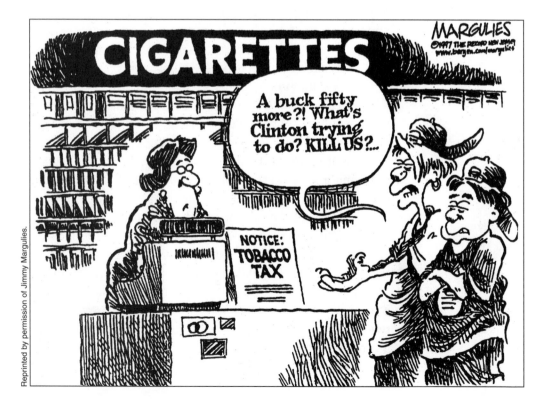

ID is now required for young people to purchase tobacco, and retailers face a $250 fine every time they are caught selling to a minor.

How do young people view stricter controls on tobacco sales? They "strongly support" a nationwide ban on tobacco, says the Gallup report. "Sixty-two percent would vote for a total ban on tobacco sales to people of all ages." Another 14 percent support a ban on sales to those under twenty-one. Among all teens, those who smoke and those who don't, 85 percent favor no sales to kids under eighteen. Surprisingly, notes Gallup, even among teen smokers, "a majority (58 percent) say they would . . . ban all tobacco sales to people under 18,"[99] which would, of course, include themselves.

Cost as a reason for quitting

Enforcing such a ban on tobacco sales could mean an incredible savings to teen smokers. According to *Consumer Reports*, American teenagers under age eighteen smoke approximately 17 billion cigarettes a year. At an average cost of 10 cents per smoke, that's nearly $2 billion spent on cigarettes each year by people who are not yet old enough to purchase the product legally!

A fifteen-year-old who smokes a pack a day spends approximately $750 per year on the habit. At the end of five years, he or she has little to show for the $3,750 investment other than yellowed teeth, bad breath, reduced lung function, and a head start on premature death. If, instead, the teen smoker had invested that money at a modest 10 percent interest, at the end of five years, he/she would have accumulated nearly $5,000. Leaving that $5,000 invested at the same rate for the next forty years would result in a $238,000 nest egg by the time the nonsmoker was sixty.

But assuming that the fifteen-year-old instead becomes a lifetime smoker, buying a pack a day (and many smoke twice that), he or she will buy 14,600 packs of cigarettes in a forty-year period. Even if cigarette prices remain at approximately $2.00 per pack, the smoker will have spent nearly $30,000 on the smoking habit from age fifteen to

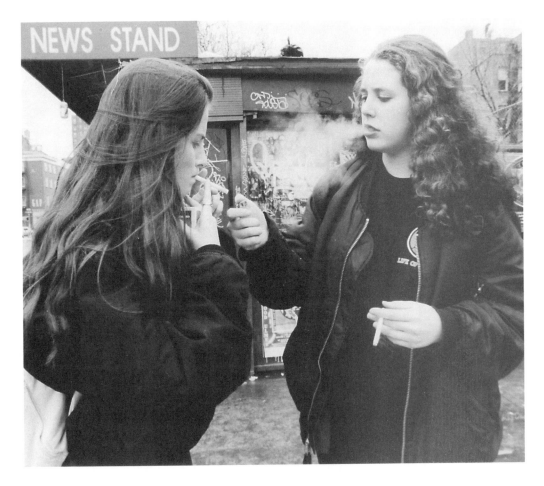

NEWS STAND

age fifty-five. And that money only buys the cigarettes. It doesn't cover the higher costs of health, car, and fire insurance that smokers pay over nonsmokers. Nor does it cover the costs to society of additional health-related expenses and days lost from work that most smokers incur because they are more prone to illness than nonsmokers.

The smoker is not the only one to lose financially because of the tobacco habit. On average, reports the Centers for Disease Control and Prevention, 7 percent of health care costs in the United States are smoking-related. For every package of cigarettes sold, the CDC estimates health care costs of $2.06—more, on average, than the price of a package of cigarettes! The cost of smoking-related health care has become a huge burden to state and federal governments.

Smoking is an expensive habit. Teens who continue smoking into adulthood will spend approximately $30,000 on cigarettes by the time they reach age fifty-five.

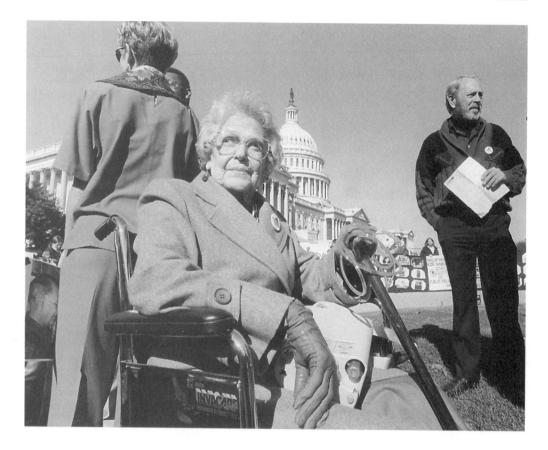

A victim of lung disease, this longtime smoker is now confined to a wheelchair and is dependent on an oxygen tank. Besides crippling the body, smoking-related illnesses can cause smokers to spend thousands of dollars in health care costs throughout their lives.

The burden has prompted some states to sue the tobacco companies to recover financial damages incurred in providing health care.

Take the case of Shirley, a lifelong smoker who started as a teenager. At age seventy-seven, she was hospitalized with massive cardiovascular problems that her doctors attributed to smoking. Her hospital bill was in excess of $50,000, yet Shirley herself paid only $875. Eighty percent of the remainder—approximately $39,300—was covered by Medicare, the national health care plan for the elderly that is financed by deductions from workers' salaries. The question raised by Shirley's case, and by thousands like it, is this: With Medicare suffering from a lack of funds, should it be required to bear the huge (and growing) costs of smoking-related illnesses? The tobacco industry answers rather flippantly that in the long run society comes out ahead financially, since smokers die relatively young, without draining retirement benefits or spending decades in nursing homes!

More good reasons to quit

In addition to the high cost of smoking, both in dollars and health, there are commonsense reasons to stop tobacco use. A majority of leaders in professional fields—business, sports, entertainment, politics, education—don't use tobacco products. Seeing that, teen smokers should ask themselves, "If two-thirds of teenagers and three-fourths of adults have chosen not to smoke, why is it so cool?"

Many high-profile heroes and former users are now speaking out against the evils of smoking. Recently the New Jersey Nets basketball team members and staff went so far as to run antismoking ads in their game programs and fan magazines. One-time model and magazine cover girl Janet Sackman was a seventeen-year-old nonsmoker

The Benefits of Quitting

20 minutes	after quitting, a smoker's blood pressure and pulse rate reduce to normal, as does the body temperature of his or her feet and hands.
8 hours	after quitting, carbon monoxide level drops and oxygen level rises to normal.
24 hours	after quitting, the risk of heart attack decreases.
48 hours	after quitting, a smoker's ability to taste and smell is enhanced.
2 weeks	after quitting, circulation improves, walking is easier, and breathing efficiency increases by nearly 30 percent.
1 year	after quitting, the risk of coronary disease declines by 50 percent.

when she accepted an offer to advertise for Lucky Strike cigarettes. To make her ads look more realistic, the company suggested that she begin smoking. Sixty-four years later, Janet appeared in a CNN television interview barely able to make herself understood. A lifetime of smoking had devastated her throat, resulting in the removal of her voice box. She "spoke" by projecting air through a hole in her esophagus. "I wish I had realized how important my life was when I was 17," Janet confessed. She added, "The single most important thing to do for your looks and your life, the single most important thing, is not to smoke."[100]

Many teens justify their decision to smoke by pointing to a relative who smoked all his or her life and died of natural causes in old age. Such representatives of earlier generations were fortunate to have survived a lifetime of smoking, particularly because they lacked the extensive medical knowledge now available about its harmful effects. Had they known and quit, millions of lives might have been prolonged.

Nor is the excuse "My friends all smoke" a valid reason for starting or continuing. Being the lone ranger in the midst of a crowd of smokers may be intimidating at first, but setting the right example for addicted friends can be very rewarding. Rather than using friends as a reason to continue smoking, a good friend will get the others to quit, too!

Breaking the addiction

Making the firm, irrevocable decision to quit tobacco products can be very difficult. Heroin or crack addicts and confirmed alcoholics often require medical treatment to break their addictions. Since nicotine is more addictive than other drugs, it's not surprising that merely desiring to quit is often not a strong enough inducement. In such cases, a family doctor can provide a referral for medical help or counseling.

For teens who want to quit on their own, there are step-by-step procedures to help ease the process. Hundreds of groups offer stop-smoking programs; the key to choosing one that works is to look for the plan that best fits the

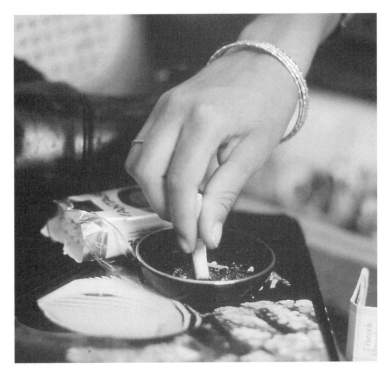

Because nicotine is a highly addictive drug, quitting smoking may take more than individual willpower. Medical treatment or counseling can help smokers break the addiction.

smoker's lifestyle. Organizations like the American Heart and American Lung Associations, and the American Cancer Society publish flyers and offer advice to aid quitters. The Quit Smoking Company, based in Georgia, is a clearinghouse for dozens of products and publications designed to help people quit tobacco.

The National Institutes of Health (NIH) publishes a list on the Internet with helpful tips and other information called "Clearing the Air: How to Quit Smoking . . . and Quit for Keeps." Once users have made the decision to quit, advises NIH, they should prepare themselves psychologically. This involves recognizing, but not dwelling on, the fact that quitting will be difficult. They must educate themselves about withdrawal, so they know what to expect as the body adjusts to the absence of nicotine. This will give them courage when the initial stages of withdrawal leave them feeling worse than they've felt in a long time.

It helps to set a target date for quitting, rather than promising to do it "soon." Once the target date has been set, NIH advises writing a list of personal reasons for quitting, such as "to please my girlfriend." Quitters should keep this list handy to reread as often as necessary when willpower lags. It helps to involve another person in the quitting process, not necessarily another tobacco user. That person can give moral support when the going gets tough, as it will.

Next, quitters must begin conditioning themselves. To help offset the negative effects of withdrawal, NIH advises getting plenty of sleep each night, drinking lots of nonalcoholic fluids, exercising regularly, and avoiding fatigue. In preparation for quitting, users should switch to a more distasteful brand, particularly one lower in tar and nicotine. Making tobacco use unpleasant is an important step in quitting. Spitting into or collecting butts in a glass jar is a very graphic way of reminding oneself just how disgusting tobacco really is.

In preparing to break the addiction, quitters should stop using tobacco out of habit—smoke or chew only when the craving becomes intolerable. One way to do this is to put cigarettes or chew in an inconvenient location. Storing tobacco products in another building, or keeping none on hand, is a great way to cut down! Finally, suggests NIH, "Don't think [about] *never* smoking again. Think of quitting in terms of *1 day at a time*. Tell yourself you won't smoke today and then, don't." [101]

Staying tobacco-free

"Clearing the Air" also offers tips on how to stay tobacco-free, after the initial withdrawal period has passed. Rule one is to throw away all tobacco products. Having none around makes it difficult to yield to temptation. Quitters should stay away from places or situations where they once used tobacco. If smokers gather beside the "tobacco-free zone" signs outside school, stay away. Being around tobacco fumes renews the nicotine urge.

Because alcohol and coffee are often associated with smoking, they should be avoided. Both are harmful to one's health, so avoiding them is beneficial in multiple ways. NIH advises finding low-calorie substitutes such as diet and caffeine-free drinks, natural juices, and water that will satisfy the oral craving. Drinking a glass of water just before meals or when hungry can help avoid weight gain, since water gives a full feeling without adding calories.

Often, smokers say they pick up a cigarette when they don't know what to do with their hands. Carrying some small object like a worry stone that can be handled during anxious moments helps to relieve this need. If the urge does become overwhelming, says NIH, try deep breathing. This relaxes the body, supplies additional oxygen to the brain, and allows the anxiety of nicotine withdrawal to pass without eating, drinking, or succumbing to the urge. Establishing daily routines is also helpful. Because exercise is so important, NIH advises quitters to choose a form they enjoy—working out at a gym, running, swimming, bicycling—and to do it faithfully on a daily basis.

Graduates of a smoking withdrawal program run by the American Cancer Society. Such programs help smokers overcome their habit by teaching them about the difficult process of nicotine withdrawal.

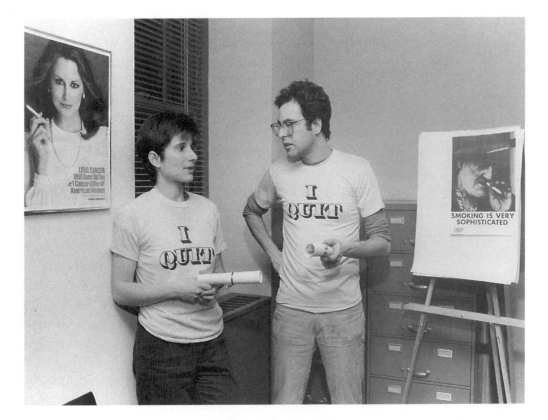

Finally, advises NIH, "Never allow yourself to think that 'one won't hurt'—it will."[102] Quitters must continually say "no" to themselves. But there also comes a time to say "yes." That is after the first day, week, month, year, of being smoke-free. Successful quitters should give themselves a little reward—a special movie, a day of skiing, a concert, a hike—something fun and affordable. It's important that quitters reward their achievement, to give themselves the incentive to stay smoke-free.

Educating people on the hazards of tobacco

Quitting tobacco use is much harder than saying "no" to it in the first place. Teens who never start smoking never have to endure the agonies of quitting. But in order for teens to say "no," they must be educated about the hazards of tobacco use. Thus far, antitobacco education has been done primarily by special interest groups, in school health classes, and in classroom programs such as Drug Abuse Resistance Education, or DARE. Overall, kids report a positive reaction to these programs. An estimated 60 percent have some classroom exposure to antismoking topics each year. A like number—including four out of ten teens who do smoke—say they would gladly contribute time to tobacco education and prevention programs.

Each year the Campaign for Tobacco-Free Kids rewards youth leaders who are making outstanding contributions to tobacco education. A committee selects one national and five regional winners. Selections are based on the young people's initiative, leadership, creative thinking and problem-solving abilities, effectiveness in communicating ideas, and impact of their actions on state and local groups dealing with youth access to tobacco.

One recent national winner was fifteen-year-old Anna Markee from Tacoma, Washington, who is an officer in the local group SMOOTH: Students Mobilizing Others Out of Tobacco Habits. Anna led her classmates in documenting tobacco advertising in her town and played a vital role in the passage of a "Truth in Tobacco Advertising" resolution to restrict outdoor advertising in Tacoma. Says Anna:

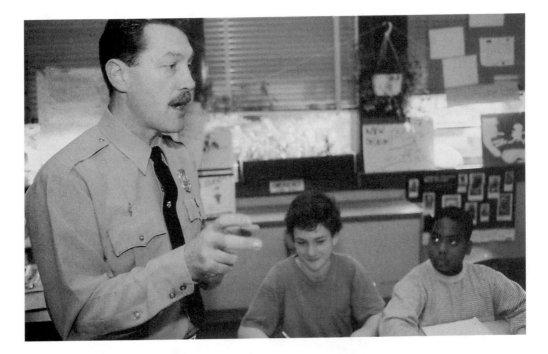

There is no single solution to the problem of teen tobacco use. . . . We need a comprehensive plan to control the amount and content of [advertising] images teens see. We need to control the amount of nicotine put in cigarettes. We need more stringent laws making it illegal to sell tobacco to minors.[103]

A DARE officer speaks to a class about tobacco and drug use. Most antismoking efforts focus on warning potential smokers of the health risks before they take up the habit.

Lara Green-Spector, a fourteen-year-old from Montclair, New Jersey, was also a winner. Lara was largely responsible for the passage of an ordinance in her town to ban both vending machines and countertop tobacco displays. Of all the antismoking projects she has helped to organize, Lara says this one was the most rewarding. "I decided to tackle this project when I saw that education and cessation programs alone would not be effective enough because cigarettes are too accessible to kids," she explained. Despite angry opposition from merchants and vending machine companies, and even opposition from the mayor, Lara held firmly to her goal. "Knowing that just one kid might not buy his/her first pack of cigarettes at a vending machine makes the long process all worth it,"[104] she says.

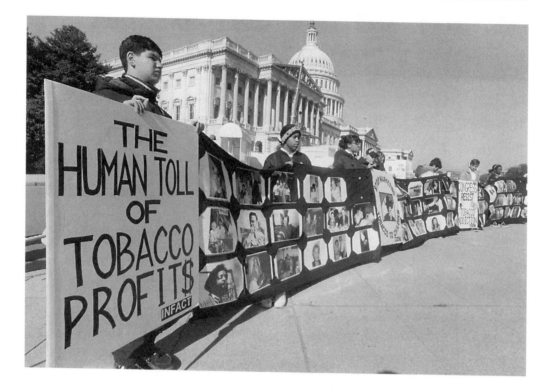

Another method of warning teens against smoking is by involving young people in efforts to stop tobacco use. Teens tend to respond better to messages coming from their peers than from adults.

As the anti–teen smoking message spreads throughout the United States, more and more groups are beginning to hold rallies and participate in local "smoke-out" days. Emily Broxterman, a Campaign for Tobacco-Free Kids award–winning ninth grader from Overland Park, Kansas, has organized many events to help educate teens against the evils of tobacco.

> I think that prevention is one important way to keep kids from starting to smoke. When I say this, I don't mean just talking about statistics and health problems associated with tobacco, but creating unusual ideas and activities, so that kids can see that you don't have to smoke to be cool.[105]

The project that Emily considers her most successful was the Smoke-Free Teens Are Rising (STAR) Rally. On STAR Rally day, an annual event since 1996, hundreds of teenagers from across Kansas gather in the capital of Topeka to show their support for a smoke-free environment. They hold mock Senate hearings and meet their legislators. There are plays and skits, and students chant antismoking slogans and messages and hear speeches by the governor, state attorney general, and other officials. So popular has the event become, says Emily, that "schools [are] actually fighting each other to come. Just watching the enthusiasm and excitement the teens had for this issue and seeing the impact the rally had on them was very rewarding."[106]

In the end, these teen leaders agree, there is nothing one teenager can do to make another one quit using tobacco. The motivation and the desire to quit must come from the user. Noel Reynolds, a college freshman from South Carolina, has a brother who is a smoker. Says Noel,

> If I knew what to say to make him stop, believe me I would tell him. We are friends and I have talked to him (not lectured) about the harmful effects of tobacco. I constantly remind him of how bad it is and I will not support his habit. However, I also tell him I am there for him if he wants to quit. All I can do is be his friend. The decision to quit is his to make, and when he chooses to make it, I will help him.[107]

Emily prefers to focus her attention on prevention rather than cessation (quitting). "It will be much harder . . . to get these teens to stop than it would be to prevent them from starting in the first place,"[108] she points out.

Anna, too, admits that fighting teen tobacco addiction can be an uphill road:

> Every once in a while I feel like this cause is hopeless or that no one cares about what I am doing. I always try to remember why I do what I do, not for recognition or support but to save lives. I never stay discouraged for long. I am constantly reminded of the problem of teen smoking.[109]

Lara takes a more long-term view, focusing on a broad-based attitude change as the force that will eventually stem the tide of teen tobacco use:

> The single most effective way to keep teenagers from becoming tobacco users is to change the beliefs and customs of society. To make tobacco use socially unacceptable is the ultimate goal of the anti-smoking message.[110]

Notes

Introduction

1. Interview with the author in Boulder County, Colorado, January 1998.

2. Quoted in Susan S. Lang and Beth H. Marks, *Teens and Tobacco: A Fatal Attraction.* New York: Twenty-First Century Books, 1996, p. 88.

3. Quoted in Lynn Minton, "Fresh Voices," *Parade Magazine*, February 1, 1998, p. 18.

4. Quoted in Campaign for Tobacco-Free Kids Factsheets, "New Evidence Supports FDA Proposal." Washington, DC: National Center for Tobacco-Free Kids, 1997.

5. Quoted in Lang and Marks, *Teens and Tobacco*, p. 12.

6. Quoted in Lang and Marks, *Teens and Tobacco*, p. 116.

7. Quoted in Campaign for Tobacco-Free Kids Factsheets, "Smokeless Tobacco and Kids." Washington, DC: National Center for Tobacco-Free Kids, 1997.

8. Quoted in Campaign for Tobacco-Free Kids Factsheets, "Smokeless Tobacco and Kids."

9. Quoted in Lang and Marks, *Teens and Tobacco*, p. 56.

10. Quoted in STAT Fact Sheets, "Tobacco as a Gateway Drug." Springfield, MA: STAT (Stop Teenage Addiction to Tobacco), 1997.

11. STAT Fact Sheets, "Tobacco as a Gateway Drug."

12. Quoted in STAT Fact Sheets, "Tobacco as a Gateway Drug."

13. Campaign for Tobacco-Free Kids Factsheets, "Tobacco and Other Drugs." Washington, DC: National Center for Tobacco-Free Kids, 1997.

Chapter 1: To Smoke or Not to Smoke

14. Quoted in Philip J. Hilts, *Smoke Screen: The Truth Behind the Tobacco Industry Cover-Up.* Reading, MA: Addison-Wesley, 1996, p. 63.

15. Quoted in Lang and Marks, *Teens and Tobacco*, p. 31.

16. Lang and Marks, *Teens and Tobacco*, p. 31.

17. Robert Bezilla, "The Spiral of Teen-Age Tobacco Addiction," *Report on the George H. Gallup International Institute's Study of Teen-Age Attitudes and Behavior Concerning Tobacco*, October 9, 1993, Summary.

18. Interview with the author in Boulder County, Colorado, January 1998.

19. Interview with the author in Jefferson County, Colorado, January 1998.

20. Quoted in Lang and Marks, *Teens and Tobacco*, pp. 56–57.

21. Quoted in Minton, "Fresh Voices," p. 18.

22. Interview with the author in Boulder County, Colorado, January 1998.

23. Interview with the author in Boulder County, Colorado, January 1998.

24. Interview with the author in Boulder County, Colorado, January 1998.

25. Interview with the author in Boulder County, Colorado, January 1998.

26. Interview with the author in Boulder County, Colorado, January 1998.

27. State of Washington, "Tobacco Facts: The Human Costs." State of Washington, 1997. Available on-line: www.wa.gov/ago/tobacco/tobacco_facts. html

28. Interview with the author in Boulder County, Colorado, January 1998.

Chapter 2: The Frightening Truth About Tobacco Addiction

29. Quoted in Laurie Kellman, "Tobacco Executives Wiggle on Question of Addiction," *Rocky Mountain News*, February 25, 1998, p. 34A.

30. Quoted in Hilts, *Smoke Screen*, p. 64.

31. Interview with the author in Boulder County, Colorado, January 1998.

32. Quoted in Hilts, *Smoke Screen*, pp. 71, 73.

33. Lang and Marks, *Teens and Tobacco*, p. 35.

34. *Random House Webster's Dictionary*, 2nd ed.

35. Quoted in Hilts, *Smoke Screen*, p. 50.

36. Interview with the author in Boulder County, Colorado, January 1998.

37. Bezilla, "The Spiral of Teen-Age Tobacco Addiction," Summary.

38. Quoted in Lang and Marks, *Teens and Tobacco*, p. 34.

39. Carl E. Bartecchi, Thomas D. MacKenzie, and Robert W. Schrier, "The Global Tobacco Epidemic," *Scientific American*, May 1995, p. 46.

40. Interview with the author in Boulder County, Colorado, January 1998.

41. Quoted in Lang and Marks, *Teens and Tobacco*, p. 34.

42. Quoted in Lang and Marks, *Teens and Tobacco*, p. 71.

43. Quoted in Lang and Marks, *Teens and Tobacco*, p. 71.

Chapter 3: Dying a Slow Death

44. Campaign for Tobacco-Free Kids Factsheets, "Tobacco Use Among Youth." Washington, DC: National Center for Tobacco-Free Kids, 1997.

45. Interview with the author in Boulder County, Colorado, January 1998.

46. Interview with the author in Boulder County, Colorado, January 1998.

47. Campaign for Tobacco-Free Kids Factsheets, "Restricting Tobacco Ads That Appeal to Children." Washington, DC: National Center for Tobacco-Free Kids, 1997.

48. Quoted in Barbara S. Lynch and Richard J. Bonnie, eds., *Growing Up Tobacco Free: Preventing Nicotine Addiction in Children and Youths*. Washington, DC: National Academy Press, 1994, p. 8.

49. Quoted in Jeff Jacoby, "Tobacco Jihad All About Power," *Rocky Mountain News*, March 28, 1998, p. 60A.

50. Interview with the author in Boulder County, Colorado, January 1998.

51. Factsheets on Teenage Cigarette Smoking, "Teenage Girls as the Target of the Tobacco Industry." Washington, DC: American Lung Association, 1997.

52. Quoted in Lang and Marks, *Teens and Tobacco*, p. 68.

53. Campaign for Tobacco-Free Kids Factsheets, "Smoking and Kids." Washington, DC: National Center for Tobacco-Free Kids, 1997.

54. "Stroke Prevention: Reducing Risk and Recognizing Symptoms." Englewood, CO: National Stroke Association, 1994.

55. Quoted in Lang and Marks, *Teens and Tobacco*, p. 66.

56. Interview with the author in Boulder County, Colorado, January 1998.

57. Quoted in Campaign for Tobacco-Free Kids Factsheets, "African Americans and Smoking." Washington, DC: National Center for Tobacco-Free Kids, 1997.

58. Quoted in Campaign for Tobacco-Free Kids Factsheets, "African Americans and Smoking."

59. Interview with the author in Boulder County, Colorado, January 1998.

60. Quoted in STAT (Stop Teenage Addiction to Tobacco), "Black Youth Are the Next Target for RJR," *Tobacco-Free Youth Reporter*, vol. 9, no. 1, March 1997, p. 3.

61. STAT (Stop Teenage Addiction to Tobacco), "Black Youth," *Tobacco-Free Youth Reporter*, p. 3.

Chapter 4: Targeting Teens

62. C. Everett Koop, David C. Kessler, and George D. Lundberg, "Reinventing American Tobacco Policy," *Journal of the American Medical Association*, February 18, 1998, pp. 550–51.

63. Quoted in Cheryl Clark, "Advertising, Teen Smoking Found Related," *San Diego Union-Tribune*, February 18, 1998, p. A-1.

64. Hilts, *Smoke Screen*, p. 65.

65. Quoted in Campaign for Tobacco-Free Kids Factsheets, "FDA Rule-at-a-Glance." Washington, DC: National Center for Tobacco-Free Kids, 1997.

66. Quoted in Campaign for Tobacco-Free Kids Factsheets, "Smokeless Tobacco and Kids."

67. Hilts, *Smoke Screen*, p. 65.

68. Quoted in Hilts, *Smoke Screen*, p. 67.

69. Bezilla, "The Spiral of Teen-Age Tobacco Addiction," Summary.

70. Quoted in Campaign for Tobacco-Free Kids Factsheets, "Smoking and Kids."

71. Campaign for Tobacco-Free Kids Factsheets, "Tobacco Marketing Attracts Kids." Washington, DC: National Center for Tobacco-Free Kids, 1997.

72. Bezilla, "The Spiral of Teen-Age Tobacco Addiction," Summary.

73. Interview with the author in Boulder County, Colorado, January 1998.

74. Lang and Marks, *Teens and Tobacco*, p. 47.

75. Interview with the author in Boulder County, Colorado, January 1998.

76. Bezilla, "The Spiral of Teen-Age Tobacco Addiction," Summary.

77. Campaign for Tobacco-Free Kids Factsheets, "Restricting Tobacco Ads That Appeal To Children." Washington, DC: National Center for Tobacco-Free Kids, 1997.

Chapter 5: The Big Winners

78. Stanton A. Glantz, John Slade, Lisa A. Bero, Peter Hanauer, and Deborah E. Barnes, *The Cigarette Papers*. Berkeley and Los Angeles: University of California Press, 1996, p. 13.

79. Quoted in Hilts, *Smoke Screen*, p. 68.

80. Patrick Reynolds and Tom Shachtman, *The Gilded Leaf: Triumph, Tragedy and Tobacco—Three Generations of the R. J. Reynolds Family and Fortune*. Boston: Little, Brown, 1989, p. 87.

81. Hilts, *Smoke Screen*, p. 2.

82. Hilts, *Smoke Screen*, p. 5.

83. Quoted in Glantz et al., *The Cigarette Papers*, p. 2.

84. Quoted in Campaign for Tobacco-Free Kids Factsheets, "New Evidence Supports FDA Proposal." Washington, DC: National Center for Tobacco-Free Kids, 1997.

85. Quoted in Campaign for Tobacco-Free Kids Factsheets, "New Evidence Supports FDA Proposal."

86. Quoted in Lang and Marks, *Teens and Tobacco*, p. 111.

87. Quoted in Borgna Brunner, ed., *Information Please Almanac*. Boston: Information Please LLC, 1998, p. 605.

88. Quoted in Campaign for Tobacco-Free Kids Factsheets, "Quotes to Note." Washington, DC: National Center for Tobacco-Free Kids, 1997.

89. Quoted in Campaign for Tobacco-Free Kids Factsheets, "Quotes to Note."

90. Campaign for Tobacco-Free Kids Factsheets, "FDA Rule-at-a-Glance."

91. Quoted in Jill Abramson, "Tobacco Firms Increase Gifts," *Rocky Mountain News*, March 8, 1998, p. 34A.

92. Koop, Kessler, and Lundberg, "Reinventing American Tobacco Policy," p. 550.

93. Quoted in Brunner, *Information Please Almanac*, p. 605.

94. Quoted in Michael Romano, "Teen Takes a Stand in Congress," *Rocky Mountain News*, March 20, 1998, p. 5A.

Chapter 6: When it's OK to Be a Quitter

95. Bezilla, "The Spiral of Teen-Age Tobacco Addiction," Summary.

96. Lang and Marks, *Teens and Tobacco*, p. 12.

97. Bezilla, "The Spiral of Teen-Age Tobacco Addiction," Summary.

98. Bezilla, "The Spiral of Teen-Age Tobacco Addiction," Summary.

99. Bezilla, "The Spiral of Teen-Age Tobacco Addiction," Summary.

100. Quoted in Lang and Marks, *Teens and Tobacco*, p. 51.

101. National Institutes of Health, "Clearing the Air: How to Quit Smoking . . . and Quit for Keeps." Alpharetta, GA: Quit Smoking Company, 1997. Available on-line: www.quitsmoking.com/quitinfo.htm.

102. National Institutes of Health, "Clearing the Air."

103. Written interview with the author through the Campaign for Tobacco-Free Kids, April 1998.

104. Written interview with the author through the Campaign for Tobacco-Free Kids, April 1998.

105. Written interview with the author through the Campaign for Tobacco-Free Kids, April 1998.

106. Written interview with the author through the Campaign for Tobacco-Free Kids, April 1998.

107. Written interview with the author through the Campaign for Tobacco-Free Kids, April 1998.

108. Written interview with the author through the Campaign for Tobacco-Free Kids, April 1998.

109. Written interview with the author through the Campaign for Tobacco-Free Kids, April 1998.

110. Written interview with the author through the Campaign for Tobacco-Free Kids, April 1998.

Glossary

addiction: The process of becoming physiologically dependent on a drug; when the process is complete, the person's state is also called addiction.

advocate, advocacy groups: A person (or group of people) who actively and publicly supports a cause or goal.

carbon monoxide: CO, an odorless, colorless gas given off as a cigarette burns; when inhaled, CO attaches itself to the body's red blood cells, depriving a person of oxygen.

cardiovascular: Pertaining to the heart and blood vessels.

CDC: Centers for Disease Control and Prevention, an agency of the federal government within the Department of Health and Human Services, made up of eleven centers, whose mission is to prevent and control disease, injury, and disability in the United States.

coronary heart disease: Diseases of the heart, specifically those that affect the supply of blood to the heart muscle; often associated with heart attacks.

dependency: The state of being physically or psychologically in need of a drug or other addictive substance.

emphysema: A chronic lung disease, often associated with smoking, that causes the air passages to lose their elastic quality, making breathing progressively more difficult.

epidemic: A disease or other health-related condition that affects many individuals at the same time.

ETS: Environmental tobacco smoke, both mainstream and sidestream smoke, put into the air by smokers.

FDA: The U.S. Food and Drug Administration, an agency of the federal Department of Health and Human Services that establishes regulations to ensure that certain foods and drugs are pure and properly labeled; tobacco is not regulated by the FDA, but that may change soon.

fertility problems: Difficulties in producing offspring.

gateway drug: A drug that serves as an introduction to other, usually stronger, more harmful drugs.

habitual user: A person who uses a product regularly enough to create a consistent pattern of behavior.

impotence: The total inability of a male to perform sexually.

intoxicate: To have one's actions excited or suppressed, to have control of one's physical and mental powers diminished as a result of ingesting drugs or alcohol.

lung cancer: A malignant (harmful) growth or tumor in the lungs that tends to spread and can eventually cause death.

mainstream smoke: Smoke released when a smoker exhales.

menthol: A colorless form of alcohol extracted from peppermint oil or made synthetically, which is used in cigarettes to cool the harsh burning sensation experienced when a smoker inhales.

nicotine: A highly toxic liquid alkaloid (bitter-tasting, nitrogen-containing compound) found in tobacco.

oral cancer: A malignant (harmful) growth or tumor in the mouth or throat that tends to spread and may eventually cause death.

passive smoking: The inhaling of another person's tobacco smoke.

peer pressure: Urging or encouragement from one's equals (in age, status, etc.) to undertake a particular act.

point-of-purchase displays: Countertop or rack placement of cigarettes or other merchandise in retail stores so that they are readily visible and accessible to customers.

pulmonary diseases: Illnesses caused by malfunctioning of the lungs.

replacement smokers: New smokers, usually teenagers, that tobacco companies lure into using their products in an effort to replace customers who have quit or died.

respiratory diseases: Those that affect the breathing apparatus.

sidestream smoke: Smoke produced when a cigarette or other tobacco product is left burning.

smokeless tobacco: Any form of tobacco that is not burned, such as snuff or plug.

snuff: Powdered tobacco inhaled through the nostrils or, more commonly, placed between the cheek and the gum for absorption into the bloodstream.

starters: People who are just beginning to use tobacco products.

stroke: A blockage of blood supply to the brain, which can cause long-term impairment or death.

surgeon general: An appointed position within the Department of Health and Human Services; the surgeon general is a physician whose job is to advise the president on public health policy.

tar: A chemically complex dark, sticky material in cigarettes that gives them their flavor.

TIRC: Tobacco Industry Research Committee, an organization formed in the early 1950s by executives of the major American tobacco companies to counter reports then beginning to surface about the harmful effects of tobacco.

warning labels: Statements from the surgeon general that must be printed on all tobacco products and advertisements for those products.

withdrawal: The process of ceasing to use an addictive drug, usually associated with physical and emotional changes to a person's system.

Organizations
to Contact

Action on Smoking and Health (ASH)
2013 H St. NW
Washington, DC 20006
(202) 659-4310
Internet: www.ash.org

The nation's oldest and largest legal-action antismoking organization that protects the rights of nonsmokers.

American Cancer Society
(800) ACS-2345
Internet: www.cancer.org

With 3,400 offices nationwide, it is the largest community-based voluntary health organization in the United States, dedicated to eliminating cancer as a major health problem through research, education, advocacy, and service. Publishes much educational material and sponsors youth involvement projects to increase awareness about the causes and preventive methods for dealing with cancer. For more information, call the toll-free number or visit the ACS website for your local office.

American Lung Association
(800)-LUNG-USA
Internet: www.lungusa.org

National organization whose mission is to prevent lung disease and promote lung health. Publishes many periodicals, brochures, and educational materials. Call or visit their website for specific information or local addresses in your area.

Campaign for Tobacco-Free Kids

1707 L St. NW, Suite 800
Washington, DC 20036
(202) 296-5469 • (800) 284-KIDS
Internet: www.tobaccofreekids.org

The country's largest nongovernment initiative to protect children from tobacco addiction. Works to protect kids from tobacco through a variety of educational programs, youth advocate awards, sponsorship of tobacco-free awareness events such as Kick Butts Day, and other national and grassroots activities. For more information on national Kick Butts Day, go to www.kickbuttsday.org.

Imperial Cancer Research Fund

Internet: www.lif.icnet.uk

British-based charity dedicated to saving lives through research into the causes, prevention, treatment, and cure of cancer. Undertakes over one-third of all cancer research in the United Kingdom. Has a section on its website called "Kids' Stuff."

Quit Smoking Company

1327 Preakness Dr.
Alpharetta, GA 30202
(770) 642-5520
e-mail: webmaster@quitsmoking.com • Internet: www. quit-smoking.com/index.html

Publishes, produces, and sells a number of products to help smokers quit, including books, magazines, CD-ROMs, audio- and videotapes, pamphlets and more.

STAT (Stop Teenage Addiction to Tobacco)

511 East Columbus Ave.
Springfield, MA 01105-2556
(413) 732-7828
Internet: www.stat.org

An advocacy organization with a mission to end childhood and teenage addiction to tobacco. It is deeply involved in the tobacco wars to adopt a meaningful tobacco policy to protect the nation's health. Publishes the periodical *Tobacco-Free Youth Reporter* and many books, products, and educational tools to combat teen tobacco use, and coordinates a variety of youth involvement activities.

Youth Media Network
17872 Moro Rd.
Prunedale, CA 93907
(408) 663-9208
e-mail: Ymedia@ix.netcom.com • Internet: www.ymn.org

A health information wire service for youth that addresses real-life problems in youth-oriented ways. Provides information about tobacco use, both smoking and chewing. Encourages young people to communicate health messages through the media and to take action against the tobacco industry.

Suggestions for Further Reading

Books

Arlene B. Hirschfelder and Arlene S. Hirsch, *Kick Butts: A Kid's Guide to a Tobacco-Free America*. Morristown, NJ: Silver Burdett Press, 1988. A 160-page book for young adults that not only addresses the hazards of smoking, but offers ideas and suggestions for reducing or eliminating the problem of tobacco use in this country.

Elizabeth Keyishian, *Everything You Need to Know About Smoking*. New York: Rosen, 1997. Presents the perils and problems of smoking for a teenage audience, written at a simplified reading level. Lists helpful organizations to contact.

Susan S. Lang and Beth H. Marks, *Teens and Tobacco: A Fatal Attraction*. New York: Twenty-First Century Books, 1996. Excellent book for teen readers that offers an in-depth look at why kids start smoking, how the tobacco companies lure them, and what the government is doing to curb teen tobacco use, and examines the health care crisis precipitated by tobacco.

Daniel McMillan, *Teen Smoking: Understanding the Risks*. Springfield, NJ: Enslow, 1998. Focuses on the health risks associated with tobacco use, tactics employed by tobacco manufacturers, social consequences of smoking, prevention efforts, and treatment options.

Andrew Tobias, *Kids Say Don't Smoke*. New York: Workman, 1991. Presents winning posters from the New

York City Smoke-Free Contest submitted by kids from kindergarten to twelfth grade, with enlightening commentary on the subject.

Charles F. Wetherall, *Quit for Teens: Read This Book and Stop Smoking*. Kansas City, MO: Andrews & McMeel, 1995. Shaped like a pack of cigarettes, this book offers no-nonsense facts, tips, and insights about why teens smoke and how they might stop.

Electronic Resources

Campaign for Tobacco-Free Kids Factsheets. Washington, DC: National Center for Tobacco-Free Kids, 1997. Available on-line: www.tobaccofreekids.org/html/factsheets1.cfm

Factsheets on Teenage Cigarette Smoking, "Teenage Girls as the Target of the Tobacco Industry." Washington, DC: American Lung Association, 1997. Available on-line: www.lungusa.org

Kids Campaigns, "Children and Tobacco: The Facts." Washington, DC: Benton Foundation, 1997. Available on-line: www.kidscampaigns.org/Whoseside/Parenting/tobaccofacts1.html

MORI Survey, "Teenage Smokers: Love Holds the Key." United Kingdom: Imperial Cancer Research Fund, 1996. Available on-line: www.lif.icnet.uk/news/teensmok.html

National Institutes of Health, "Clearing the Air: How to Quit Smoking . . . and Quit for Keeps." Alpharetta, GA: Quit Smoking Company, 1997. Available on-line: www.quitsmoking.com/quitinfo.htm

State of Washington, "Tobacco Facts: The Human Costs." State of Washington, 1997. Available on-line: www.wa.gov/ago/tobacco/tobacco_facts.html

State Tobacco Information Center, "Tobacco and Kids Factsheets." Boston: Tobacco Newslinks, 1997. Available on-line: http://stic.neu.edu/News/newslinks.html

"Tobacco Control Resource Center, Inc. & The Tobacco Products Liability Project." Boston: Northeastern University School of Law, 1998. Available on-line: www.tobacco.neu.edu/

"Youth and Tobacco Factsheets." Berkeley, CA: Americans for Nonsmokers' Rights, 1996. Available on-line: www.no-smoke.org/youth.html

Youth Media Network, "Tobacco Facts." Prunedale, CA: Central Coast Tobacco-Free Regional Project, 1997. Available on-line: www.ymn.org

Works Consulted

Books

Borgna Brunner, ed., *Information Please Almanac.* Boston: Information Please LLC, 1998.

Stanton A. Glantz, John Slade, Lisa A. Bero, Peter Hanauer, and Deborah E. Barnes, *The Cigarette Papers.* Berkeley and Los Angeles: University of California Press, 1996.

Philip J. Hilts, *Smoke Screen: The Truth Behind the Tobacco Industry Cover-Up.* Reading, MA: Addison-Wesley, 1996.

Barbara S. Lynch, and Richard J. Bonnie, eds., *Growing Up Tobacco Free: Preventing Nicotine Addiction in Children and Youths.* Washington, DC: National Academy Press, 1994.

Milton Moskowitz, *Everybody's Business: A Field Guide to the 400 Leading Companies in America.* New York: Doubleday, 1990.

National Stroke Association, *The Road Ahead: A Stroke Recovery Guide.* Englewood, CO: National Stroke Association, 1992.

Patrick Reynolds and Tom Shachtman, *The Gilded Leaf: Triumph, Tragedy and Tobacco—Three Generations of the R. J. Reynolds Family and Fortune.* Boston: Little, Brown, 1989.

Periodicals and Reports

Jill Abramson, "Tobacco Firms Increase Gifts," *Rocky Mountain News*, March 8, 1998.

Carl E. Bartecchi, Thomas D. MacKenzie, and Robert W. Schrier, "The Global Tobacco Epidemic," *Scientific American*, May 1995.

Robert Bezilla, "The Spiral of Teen-Age Tobacco Addiction," *Report on the George H. Gallup International Institute's Study of Teen-Age Attitudes and Behavior Concerning Tobacco*, October 9, 1993.

Cheryl Clark, "Advertising, Teen Smoking Found Related," *San Diego Union-Tribune*, February 18, 1998.

Consumer Reports, "Hooked on Tobacco: The Teen Epidemic," March 1995.

Jeff Jacoby, "Tobacco Jihad All About Power," *Rocky Mountain News*, March 28, 1998.

Laurie Kellman, "Tobacco Executives Wiggle on Question of Addiction," *Rocky Mountain News*, February 25, 1998.

Lawrence L. Knutson, "Gore Backs Higher Cost for Tobacco," *Rocky Mountain News*, March 23, 1998.

C. Everett Koop, David C. Kessler, and George D. Lundberg, "Reinventing American Tobacco Policy," *Journal of the American Medical Association*, February 18, 1998.

Lynn Minton, "Fresh Voices," *Parade Magazine*, February 1, 1998.

Michael Romano, "Teen Takes a Stand in Congress," *Rocky Mountain News*, March 20, 1998.

STAT Fact Sheets, "Tobacco as a Gateway Drug." Springfield, MA: STAT (Stop Teenage Addiction to Tobacco), 1997.

STAT (Stop Teenage Addiction to Tobacco), *Tobacco-Free Youth Reporter*, vol. 9, no. 1, March 1997.

"Stroke Prevention: Reducing Risk and Recognizing Symptoms." Englewood, CO: National Stroke Association, 1994.

Index

Picture Credits

About the Author

Eleanor H. Ayer is the author of more than fifty books for children and young adults, in the areas of history, biography, and teenage social issues. Among her titles of current interest to teens are *It's Okay to Say No: Choosing Sexual Abstinence, Homeless Children, Teen Marriage, Teen Fatherhood, Stress, Depression,* and *Teen Suicide.* Ms. Ayer earned a master's degree in literacy journalism from Syracuse University's Newhouse School of Journalism. She is survived by her husband and two sons.

		DATE DUE	